The Art of
Pulse Diagnosis

The ART of PULSE DIAGNOSIS

A STEP-BY-STEP EXPLORATION
OF METHOD, DIRECTIONALITY,
ORGAN ENERGETICS,
COMPLEMENT CHANNEL PULSES,
TEXTURES, AND IMAGES

Ann Cecil-Sterman, MS, L.Ac.

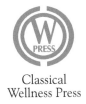

Classical
Wellness Press

The teachings in this book come through my filter from the oral tradition
through the gracious generosity of my principal teacher, Daoist Master, Dr Jeffrey Yuen.
Any mistakes are mine. A.C.S.

Cover design, book design, graphic design and diagrams: Cody Dodo
Art Copy Work: Cameron Neilson, New York.
(Additional work by Simon Shiff, Australia, pp. x and 200.)
Paintings: Ann Cecil-Sterman

ISBN: 978-0-9837720-1-9

BY THE SAME AUTHOR

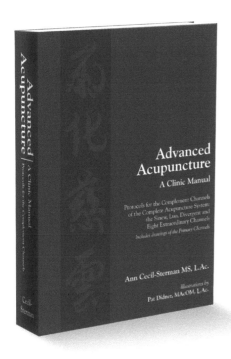

Advanced Acupuncture, A Clinic Manual
Protocols for the Complement Channels of the
Complete Acupuncture System: the Sinew, Luo, Divergent
and Eight Extraordinary Channels

Classical Wellness Press, 2012

Currently a required or recommended text in many acupuncture schools in
the USA, Europe and Australia.

Illustrations of the Complete Acupuncture System:
the Sinew, Luo, Divergent, Eight Extraordinary
and Primary Channels

Classical Wellness Press, 2014.

(This is a companion volume to *Advanced Acupuncture, A Clinic Manual*
and is not a stand-alone book. It's designed to make the Manual's
illustrations easily accessible in ring-bound form.)

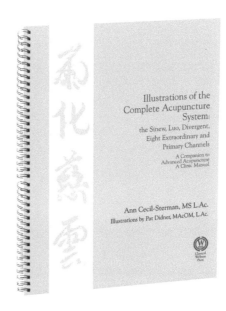

To Andrew, my partner in life and collaborator in thought.

When the book arrived it was received the way a painting arrives in the mind of the painter, and in the way it is received by those who look at the painting. Seen to be made. Witnessed, the way the branch witnesses the bird who is landing. Receptive. An urn, a chalice like space opened in the mouth and the words poured forth through the arm, painted. Painting and painted and received. Written and writing and witnessed. The book was the book it became. It became the book. A cavern. A space opened and we were written. Writing and written, the singing was hidden. We touched the book. We had been listening. The listening which became the writing, the breathing. Its perching and visiting turned to imprint. The space of the book, a permutation. A visitation. In the book there is feeling.

—Martha Oatis, 2016.

Table of Contents

List of Paintings

FOREWORD

It's easy to love books and Ann Cecil-Sterman makes it easy to love this book, *The Art of Pulse Diagnosis*. Writing for colleagues and students, Cecil-Sterman sets out to share her years of experience and knowledge about the pulses. She draws from Wang Shu He's Pulse Classic as well as the interpretation of her teacher, Jeffrey Yuen, 88th generation Daoist priest in the Jade Purity tradition. The beauty of the book comes from Cecil-Sterman's long familiarity and cultivation of the pulses in practice, as a teacher, and now as an artist. On each page one feels the joy of the technique and the wonder of its complexity.

Books, however, have limitations. The promise and potential they offer can remain enticingly out of reach. The Dao De Jing states "The Dao that can be spoken is not the true Dao." Right away, the words warn us about words. The tradition that Cecil-Sterman practices is an oral Daoist tradition which centers around the connection between the teacher and the student. While the words are the vehicle of knowledge, the transmission is seen as a deeper process. The student can receive the information for which they are ready, depending on their cultivation. Dui (hexagram 58) of the Yi Jing has this commentary on the image: "Knowledge should be a refreshing and vitalizing force. It becomes so only through stimulating intercourse with congenial friends with whom one holds discussion and practices application of the truths of life. In this way learning becomes many-sided and takes on a cheerful lightness, whereas there is always something ponderous and one–sided about the learning of the self-taught." (Wilhelm translation)

Many ancient sages were wary of books. Socrates warned that they can ruin memory and carry but the image of wisdom. The words once laid down in text become static, unable to defend themselves, unable to clarify, unable to address the needs of the individual student. Socrates' remedy was to create a discourse with his students that could model thought, that could be reflected upon and engaged with. In this way a text could remain relevant as long as the reader was willing to question and explore. We each have to come to terms with our desire to have a stable foothold of knowledge while remaining connected to the freedom and spontaneity of the moment. While a book may help, we don't want to succumb to dogmatic acceptance of what is written.

Chinese medicine has its authoritative texts such as the Nei Jing, the Nan Jing, the Shang Hun Lun, the Ben Caos. We are grateful to have these insights from centuries ago. As with Socrates, many are written as dialogues—a reminder that we are students present at this discussion. In commentaries written on these texts, we see the engagement of scholars and practitioners over the centuries.

My own journey began with the study of the Western philosophical classics many years ago.

I was thrilled when I found the acupuncture program at the Swedish Institute of Oriental Medicine in New York City which was based on the Eastern classics of medicine. During my years there studying with Jeffrey Yuen and other classically trained teachers, I came to realize it was not just the books that I loved, but that they were brought to life with my teachers and colleagues. The interaction was integral.

As a student, I dutifully memorized the 28 pulses but they seemed to be a flat confirmation of a diagnosis arrived at through other means. The richness of the pulse escaped me. This changed the day I was introduced to the dynamic pulses. It brought tangibility to the theories of Chinese medicine. I could have a dialogue with the patient's Qi and Blood, the Zang and Fu, the Primary meridians and the Complement channels.

Having taught in acupuncture programs for over 12 years at both the Swedish Institute and the Pacific College of Oriental Medicine in New York City, I am delighted to see the publication of this book. Many students feel inadequate in their interpretation of the pulse and are uncertain about how to correct it. We no longer have the long apprenticeship where we could be individually directed. In *The Art of Pulse Diagnosis*, Cecil-Sterman lays out not only the physiological underpinnings of the pulses but also their relationships to each other. From this integrated approach we can connect what we are feeling in the pulse to what we are learning in theories.

But let's not forget, a pulse is a palpation and it is difficult for any book to teach a physical practice or a sensation. Here, as readers, we must be mindful. For some, the words may create a vivid image that expands upon their pulse knowledge. Others may need to engage more intimately with a teacher. As students of Chinese Medicine, whichever way we approach *The Art of Pulse Diagnosis*, all of us can keep the work alive with discussion and application.

With the pulses, Ann Cecil-Sterman has found a window into the world of the patient; the beauty and clarity she sees there guided her to write and teach. She has put together a comprehensive, clear book that invites us to have a deeper appreciation of the pulses and inspires our own cultivation. Cecil-Sterman sets us out on this fine path and reminds us that even at the end of the book we are at the beginning of a journey.

Linda Puckette, DC LAc
New York City, 2016

ACKNOWLEDGMENTS

Throughout the production of this book I've been so grateful to have a large (and growing) supportive team comprising many precious friends. Cody Dodo, whose unique background as a graphic designer and a Jeffrey Yuen-trained acupuncturist enables him to produce exactly the right diagrams. The book design is all his; I can't imagine being able to produce these books without him. Thanks for your endless patience, expertise, and friendship, Cody.

This book would not have been possible without the meticulous and expert guidance of Dr Linda Puckette. I just can't thank you enough, Linda. Thank you to the following: Andrew Sterman, who put his many endeavors aside to read draft after draft, making pertinent, perspicacious comments. Betsy Sterman, for her thoughtful corrections and advice on the use of language throughout the entire book. Marjorie and Noel Cecil for their vast teachings, especially that anything is possible. Gretchen Kreiger for her invaluable and generous support. Holly Burling for meticulously proofreading the entire book. Josephine Spilka for her invaluable feedback and treasured counsel. Gabrielle Zlotnik for caring for the book like a grandmother, for proofreading, and for the essential and time-consuming job of making the index. Hope Hathaway for again casting her eagle eye over every detail of the entire final edit.

Heartfelt thanks to Neil Bender and Philip Glass for their wise counsel. So many thanks to Stephen Nelson for curating the art and for his transformative mentoring. Very special thanks to Cameron Neilson for setting up studio in my apartment and spending a day expertly photographing the paintings. (Such a great day.) Thank you Lois Greenfield for warm support and advice. Thank you to Diane Gioioso, Evan Rabinowitz, Monica Martin, Jill Kirschen, Dar Dowling and Libbie Rice for their love and support. Ravi and Miriam Sterman for help with the index and camera. Thank you Christina Seibel, Reuben Zylberszpic, Janine and David Cecil, Chelsea Horenstein, MaryAnne Bachia, Kathleen Furlong, Mark Phillips. Thank you Simon Shiff for generously photographing the two paintings in Australia. Thanks to the following dear colleagues who agreed to read an early draft and gave suggestions: Stephen Howard, John Heuertz, Jennifer Jackson, Grace Devlin, Donna Keefe, Youngja Yoo, Mona Dinari, David Blaiwas, Theo Yang Copley and Cissy Majebe. I appreciate the generosity of Setareh Moafi, Heather Spangler, Bart Beckermann. Doug McGill for his guiding light. Tim Turco for his unique help. Phil Sanders for his deep wisdom in art and ethics. Andie Santo Pietro for her continued compassionate, searing insight. Matt Kahn for his enthusiasm for this project and his inspiring counsel. Thank you Martha Oatis for your poignant poem.

And in the center of my heart I thank my teacher, Dr Jeffrey Yuen. His teachings are vast and limitless; seeds I didn't even know he planted surprise me as they grow, seemingly spontaneously. Above all, he continuously urges all his students to make the medicine their own, to inhabit their knowledge fully. For all this I am forever grateful and inspired.

HOW TO READ THE PAINTINGS

Bean

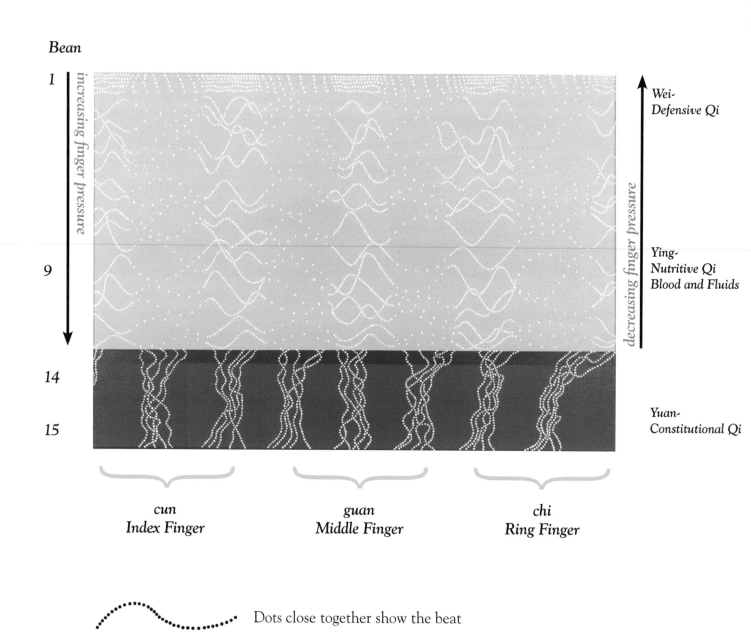

increasing finger pressure

decreasing finger pressure

1

9

14

15

Wei-
Defensive Qi

Ying-
Nutritive Qi
Blood and Fluids

Yuan-
Constitutional Qi

cun
Index Finger

guan
Middle Finger

chi
Ring Finger

Dots close together show the beat

Dots spread out show the time between beats

AUTHOR'S NOTE

In this book I am presenting segments of potent pulse practices from different eras of Chinese medicine, selected and brought together, occasionally with new or adapted nomenclature, to form a coherent working system for the way I work and teach. Pulse methods reflect the focal points of sweeping changes in the long and extraordinarily rich history of Chinese medicine. Each major clinician has looked for signs in the pulses to guide them according to their specific insights into health, illness, recovery and the thriving of their patients. For example, during the period of the Four Great Masters, Liu Wan-Su was looking for directionality and excess Heat; Zhang Zi-He was looking for the location of wiry pulses and the right time to purge; Li Dong-Yuan held both wrists at once, comparing all pulses to the Spleen/Stomach pulse; Zhu Dan-Xi related his findings to the Kidney pulses. In this context, all methodical pulse teaching is both valid and potentially risky. Taking pulses is not about ascertaining fact; it's about informing the clinical decisions central to one's way of thinking. One's pulse taking method must be in alignment and resonate with one's clinical approach. My hope is to provide some of the treasures of these traditions in a form that is highly organized and also open for expansion or selection by readers, according to their background, interests, focus, expertise and above all, personal cultivation. Rather than dictating a system, what I've organized here is material from which a practitioner could develop or hone their own clinical style.

ABOUT THE ART

When I take pulses I see large, vivid and warm-colored, moving, complex three-dimensional images. For many years I kept this to myself, then a few years ago I began to paint them. They became useful teaching tools in class discussions, as it's almost impossible to convey the feeling and texture of pulses in words. More recently, out of the office, they've become healing tools in select homes and businesses around the world. I painted the works included in this book with natural mineral pigments from different locations in Australia, my country of origin. The dot painting techniques are borrowed from the Australian Aborigines (the oldest living art tradition in the world). These artists paint the absence of separation between the viewer and the viewer's vision of the world. They celebrate that the number of ways of seeing is limitless. In my pulse paintings, these techniques enable the pulses to move, to occupy and release space, to be timeless, formless, substantial and palpable all at once. The pulse appears as a microcosm of the human landscape, timeless and boundless, full of life.

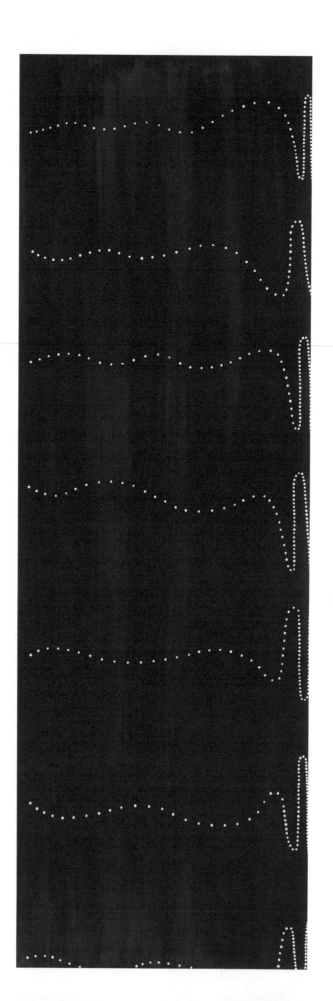

The Superficial Pulse

INTRODUCTION

The purpose of this book is to play a part in the movement to return pulse taking to its original status as the Chinese medical practitioner's principal tool of diagnosis. This book offers step-by-step protocols for pulse taking. It records in writing—possibly for the first time—the concept of Dynamic Directional Pulses.

When used to its full capacity the art of pulse taking is arguably the jewel in the crown of Chinese Medical diagnosis. It is one of the most fascinating, profound, marvelous, accurate, insightful and revealing phenomena in Chinese Medicine. With practice, in the pulse we can detect the entire gamut of pathology from the common cold to constitutional disorders and imbalances of all kinds: musculoskeletal, psychological, gastrointestinal, urogenital, reproductive, cardiovascular, respiratory, neurological, and organ disease. Past, present and future are recorded there. Bacteria, funguses and viruses. Moods, emotions and constitutional dispositions. Heat and Cold. Excesses or deficiencies of diet. The location of tension and flaccidity. The available volume and movement of each fluid.

The pulse is a window into the inseparability of body and mind. The pulses can describe to the practitioner facets of psychological history of the patient long forgotten by the patient yet still wielding long term effects on his or her unconscious mind. In the pulse one can see the origin of a disease, where it is in the body at present and where it will move to in the future. Each of the Zang Fu has a unique position in the pulse. The Primary Channels and each of the Complement Channels—the Sinew, Luo, Divergent and Eight Extraordinary Channels— are clearly mapped in the pulses. The pulses tell us which Channel to treat and the order in which to conduct the treatment. Like life itself, the information in the pulses is without limit.

The art of pulse taking as a diagnostic tool transcends the process of diagnosing by verbal dialogue and then taking the pulses to validate those findings. Simply put, the chief complaint or signs and symptoms presented are very often not the origin or root of the disease. The pulse gives us both the root and branch of the disease.

The patient might be coming to us for a sign or symptom that is an indirect result of the origin of the imbalance. For example, the patient may be suffering with headaches in the temporal region but the pulses show that the origin is not tension in the Gallbladder Channel, but weakness of the Spleen resulting in its failure to make blood. The Gallbladder hasn't enough blood to move and this is causing tightness in the Channel. In this case, diagnosing only via dialogue with the patient might lead us to treat the Gallbladder Channel, a treatment that could yield some temporary relief or may utterly fail.

Another patient, complaining about chronic bronchitis, has a long history of respiratory issues. The pulses might show that the Lungs are actually strong but that the vector between the Spleen and the Lungs is not active, so Spleen Qi is not reaching the Lungs. In this case diagnosis through dialogue would result in tonifying Lung Qi, perhaps with minimal results because it was the relationship of Spleen and Lung that needed to be treated.

Yet another patient has chronic immobilizing back pain. Then the practitioner, basing diagnosis on the verbal encounter with the patient, needles and uses moxa along the Bladder Shu line and BL-40, BL-60, etc., and is utterly confounded as to why the treatment is not holding week after week. The pulses however, show that the Heart and Kidneys are not communicating and that the diaphragm is blocked, resulting in Qi not being able to circulate to the low back from the Upper Jiao. The treatment in this case might best start at the front of the body, since communication between Heart and Kidney must be fully restored in order for Qi to be able to flow to and release the back.

In another case, the patient might be suffering night sweats. Based on the conversation, the practitioner nourishes Kidney Yin and there might be no change at all in the condition or the condition might worsen. The pulses, meanwhile, show that the Lungs are failing to descend Qi. Lung Qi must be descended in order for the night sweats to stop. Here again the pulse is a practitioner's guide to appropriate treatment choices.

The restoration of the art of pulse taking to the status of a diagnostic tool rather than one of confirmation will lead to accurate diagnoses, pertinent treatments and best of all, healthier, pleased and happy patients who report to their friends and family that acupuncture, or Chinese Medicine in general, heals. Acupuncture treats all diseases if our diagnoses are determined by a detailed systematic pulse-taking method. What matters most is that the style employed matches the style of practice and that it is used to create a detailed diagnosis.

Classical medicine is a vast field of countless styles and lineages with a corresponding variety of pulse methods. Working to share deep and comprehensive knowledge of the pulses are, for example, Will Morris, with his wonderful book, and Dr. Leon I. Hammer, who has documented a very detailed, highly developed method in his books on pulses. I urge the study of these valuable resources. The classical texts, Pulse Diagnosis by Li Shi Zhen, and especially the foundational classic, the *Mai Jing* by Wang Shu He are cornerstones of Chinese Medicine.

One of the unique features of the Manual you are about to read is the section on Directional Pulse Taking. This method involves the application and release of pressure from the radial artery. Each organ has one or several vectors: the Stomach's vector is downward, the Spleen's upward, and so on. Directional pulses give a clear reading of whether the organs are operating with their vector intact. For example, if the Stomach's vector is not in order, there will be rebellious Qi. Directional pulses give us a clear understanding of the movement of Qi throughout the body and are extremely useful in diagnosis. It's a method that is simple and easily learned. My teacher, Dr Yuen, teaches a myriad of methods and on occasion includes the aspect of Directionality. He is careful to impress that it is just one of the wide array of pulse techniques.

I have chosen to write about this aspect of pulse taking simply because in my practice I find it indispensable in the diagnosis of every one of my patients. This method is golden to me, and having included it in my teaching for many years all over the country, overseas, and especially in my own classroom, it is time to put this aspect of this vast medicine down in writing.

One of the things I enjoy most about Chinese Medicine is that it gives me the feeling of being on a lifelong journey of engaged learning. I love that. I love the feeling that no matter how hard you study and how much you apply yourself, there is no end to how much more deeply you can delve. There is no limit to the expansion of one's understanding. Pulse diagnosis is like a microcosm of the same concept. Every year, as I'm sure we all do, I discover that I can find more and more in the pulses. The strange thing is that it seems to be exponentially increasing. This is sobering. If it increases exponentially, how little does one now know? Therefore this book is not intended to be definitive; rather, it is intended as a systematic teaching of essential classical pulse diagnosis methods in a form complete enough for profound clinical application as well as opening the gate to further revelations.

I am humbled to think that this Manual may help other clinicians bring the benefits of Classical pulse-taking, and the very precise diagnoses and treatments that result, to countless patients for what can be their indescribable benefit.

May every day be one of meaningful and profound healing and wellness.

Ann Cecil-Sterman
Manhattan, 2015

NOMENCLATURE

Dynamic Pulses are pulses that require movement of the finger or fingers. Dynamic pulses have two subsets: Probing Pulses and Directional Pulses.

Directional Pulses are pulses that require the application of pressure on one pulse in order to create an effect in another pulse.

Inter-Jiao Blockages are blockages at the diaphragm or in Dai Mai. They obstruct communication between the Jiao's.

Mediumship means any fluid: Jin-Thin Fluids, Ye-Thick Fluids, Blood and Jing-Essence.

Probing Pulses are felt during an inquiry into one individual pulse using varying pressures in that pulse while the pressures applied at the other two positions remain constant.

Pulse Neutral is a term for the basic pulse taking position. The fingers at the cun and guan positions are at the moderate level and the finger at the chi position is at the deep level.

Stepped Position is a term for a pulse taking position where the finger at the cun position is at the superficial level, the finger at the guan position is at the moderate level and the finger at the chi position is at the deep level.

Static Pulses are those that are felt using no movement of the finger once the desired depth is reached.

Bean

Classically, Height is said to be measured in beans. The amount of pressure you need to apply for the pulse to yield the required information is measured in the imagined weight of mung beans. This is described in Chapter 5 of the *Mai Jing* and is figurative, of course. What really matters is the distance your finger travels relative to the total depth of the pulse. The amount of pressure required to press into the bone, occluding the flow of blood in the radial artery, is said to be 15 beans. That is a standard applied to all people, so 15 beans on one person's wrist could be several times the pressure needed on another person's.

CHAPTER 1

ORIENTATION AND DEFINITIONS

HISTORICAL CONTEXT

The principal Classical pulse text is the *Mai Jing (Pulse Treatise)*, written by Wang Shu He (180-270 CE), the great imperial physician of the later Han-Western Jing Dynasty responsible for the preservation of the *Shang Han Lun* tradition. In the Han Dynasty, acupuncture was at a pinnacle and much more sophisticated than it is today, since all the channels of the complete acupuncture system were in use. In the period spanning the Han and Tang Dynasties practitioners were well versed in the Primary and Complement channels: the Sinew, Luo, Divergent and Eight Extraordinary Channels and their corresponding pulses. The *Mai Jing* discusses static pulses and pulses that "occupy more than one position," also known as directional pulses.

Wang Shu He's book dominated until the Ming Dynasty when Li Shi Zhen (1518-1593) published his book on Pulse Diagnosis, co-authored with his father. However, by that time the use of the Sinew, Luo and Divergent Channels had gone into decline and only the Primary Channels and the Eight Extraordinary Channels were in use. Therefore Li Shi Zhen's book was based on Zang Fu, not the complete channel system, and focused mainly on 27 static pulses. At that point dynamic pulses effectively disappeared.

The current revival of the complement channels has lead to great interest in Classical pulse taking techniques. There is great interest in the pulse taking methods of the Han and Tang Dynasties. Note: My book, *Advanced Acupuncture: A Clinic Manual*, gives detailed information and clinic protocols for the application of the Sinew, Luo, Divergent and Eight Extraordinary channels.

CLASSICAL PULSE TEACHING METHOD

Classically, pulse training was one-on-one. The student would sit with the teacher as the teacher took and described pulses of a patient. The student would then compare what he himself was feeling in the patient's pulses to the teacher's findings. Today, gaining knowledge about pulses takes us on a different path, as the traditional method of one-on-one instruction is no longer feasible. Yet the classroom setting is not an ideal pulse teaching forum because the action of taking the pulse changes the pulse itself (to varying degrees). The findings of the teacher might not be felt by students beyond the first student in line to perform his or her calibration. Gathering regularly in pulse study groups is therefore invaluable practical instruction.

CULTIVATION IN PREPARATION FOR PULSE TAKING

When well versed in the art of pulse taking, the clinician is positioned to be able to see every interaction of Qi in the body. We can see not just the postnatal arena and the status of Fluids and Qi, we can see the entire constitution, the entire curriculum, the global being. The patient intuitively feels the practitioner's ability to do this. To a patient this can feel anywhere from grossly invasive to enormously exciting, depending on the attitude of the clinician. At the "invasive" end of the spectrum the patient feels that the clinician is examining the pulse at a "depth" at which he or she is not welcome, or that the clinician is overly confident, incapable of assimilating or accepting what he or she finds, or even incapable of treating what is found. The patient might intuitively feel that the practitioner will make a judgment or have an opinion about the choices made or soon to be made. Conversely, at the excitement end of the spectrum, the patient feels that the clinician is worthy of trust, very capable, experienced, calm, self-possessed, so quietly confident and solid that nothing, no emotion, no event, no aspect of the patient's personal or health history, could be surprising or shocking. Very importantly, the point where the patient places the clinician on this spectrum is directly related to the amount revealed to the clinician in the pulses, and further complicated if there is a history of trauma, cultural issues, or skepticism.

The more the patient reveals, the more accurate the diagnosis can be and the more the practitioner can be of help. If the patient cannot sense calm in the practitioner, the patient is likely to erect barriers to the clinician at the level of the pulse and close this gateway to the practitioner. Key to the posture of effective clinicians, therefore, is calm. If the patient senses peace within the practitioner, the pulses are likely allowed to communicate up to the practitioner, and with them the information they are ready to reveal in order to get the treatment that is needed. If we are genuinely internally calm and at peace within ourselves, our patients will more likely allow themselves to be fully present in the pulse. We have so many tools at the ready to help us as clinicians: daily meditation, daily qigong, daily tai ji, daily grounding time, affirmations, stones, a calming diet. Without a daily practice, a true physical union at the pulse level is very difficult.

The union of the practitioner and patient at the site of the pulse is also greatly supported when the practitioner holds the view that there is no actual separation between the two. Chapter One of the *Ling Shu* says that when you are treating an individual it is important to pay attention to the spirit of the client as well as to your own. This is asking us to examine whether we see the patient as separate from us or not. With cultivation we arrive at compassion and understand with our entire beings that there is no separation. In short, if we are calm and at peace, if we are in a state of oneness, if we understand that the pulses are a reflection of the macrocosm called earth, if we observe ourselves before we observe the pulse, and if we understand our true interconnectedness to the patient, the patient will allow those gateways to open and welcome our reception of their pulse.

In interconnectedness not only are we receiving information, we are imprinting the way the patient can overcome his or her difficulty since all difficulties arise through forgetting that we are not separate. As we remind ourselves that all apparent negativity is in the process of being transformed, the patient too is reminded and resonates that notion. So we are imparting healing through the vibrations of our intention, through the vibration of our spiritual orientation.

QIGONG OF THE PULSES

Extrapolating on the oneness of all things and the interconnectedness of all beings it's important to note that the healing process—or more accurately the invitation to heal—comes from the first touch. You could argue that it occurs with the greeting at the door, or during the communication in which the appointment was made, but let's focus on the first palpation. Classically it was considered that pulse taking was the first opportunity to encourage a patient to bring their Qi to move in a certain way. This is the first action of the practitioner's intention. When you touch the pulses and feel something "pathological" you can ask it to change. If the pulse is too fast, we can ask it to slow down, if it's too slow, we can ask it to speed up. If it's irregular, we can ask it to regulate itself. This interaction with the pulses initiates the healing process even before a diagnosis has been made, even before a single needle is inserted. The way in which we touch the pulse is equivalent to doing qigong on the channels or the organs; we are inviting the Qi to move.

MEANING OF PULSE POSITION NAMES: THE CUN, GUAN AND CHI

Chapter Three of the *Mai Jing* explains the meaning of the names of the pulse positions, the cun, guan and chi.

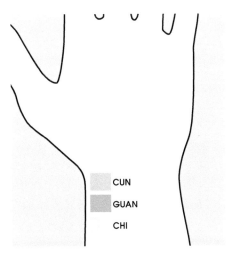

CUN

GUAN

CHI

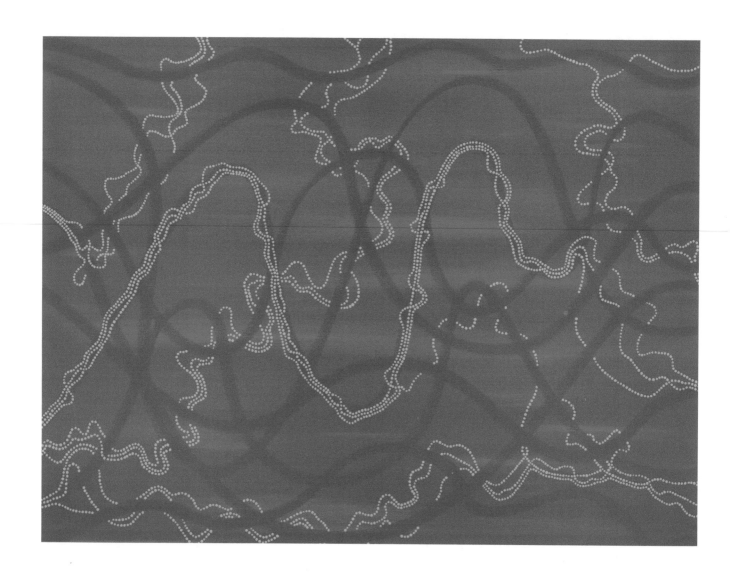

Blueprint

This painting depicts the deepest level of energetics in the body, the level of Yuan (Constitutional) Qi. This Qi is a fusion of Essence inherited from the parents and Heavenly Qi which enters at the moment of conception. Infused in this dense Qi is the blueprint for that life, including the DNA. The uniqueness of the individual's Constitutional Qi guarantees a unique life's purpose. Sometimes we traverse paths that are not part of the blueprint, resisting what we already know on a deeper level to be our true path. A true path is one of relaxed certainty.

The word cun means measurement. The art of pulse taking is the art of making measurements of the movement of Yin and Yang. The cun position is in the area of LU-9, the Qi Mouth.

The word guan means gateway. Sometimes this is translated as barrier. The Middle Jiao and in particular a healthy Spleen, is the gateway to health. The Liver is also at the guan position; the Liver is the gateway between the Upper and Lower Jiaos. It's also the gateway to various levels of consciousness, and provides entrée to the collective unconscious.

The word chi means pattern, as in a tailor's pattern or a pattern maker's design grid. Through the chi position we can see the pattern that has been laid out in the constitution, the template from which the patient's life is being played out. The themes of our lives are created from a pattern or template stored in the Jing-Essence. At any moment we are constitutionally expressing our pattern, our destiny as it stands at that moment.

The word chi also translates as 10 cun. To look into the chi pulse is to see 10 cun into the Yuan level. Clearly, the pulse cannot literally be 10 cun deep anatomically, so this refers to the possibility of seeing very deeply into the constitution, the destiny, the Will, the curriculum of that life. To be able to see to a depth of ten cun at the chi position means to be able to obtain a reading of the unlimited depth of the constitution. With practice, there's no limit to what one can discern from the chi pulse. We can even see past trauma there. If you inquire about an event that you might sense in the chi position and it becomes tight while you are talking about it, the memory of that period might be very traumatic. As practitioners we can bring these events into consciousness to enable the patient to heal from insults to the Jing-Essence. Healing is not to prevent death, but to free the patient from constraints in the passage of life.

When read together, the pulse enables us to measure (cun) movements through the gateway (guan) that is the pulse and understand the pattern (chi) that is the marked template expressing from the curriculum—the program of one's life stored in the Kidneys.

DEFINITIONS: DYNAMIC, DIRECTIONAL, PROBING AND STATIC PULSES

Dynamic pulse taking is a vast field which involves being sensitive to the way in which a pulse behaves under a moving finger. Dynamic pulse taking reveals the interrelationship of the various organs in the entire pulse grid, that is, across the three levels of energetics in the pulses (the Wei, Ying and Yuan levels) in the cun, guan and chi positions.

Directional pulses are a subset of dynamic pulses and are revealed when coordinated movements of one or more fingers create hydraulic actions in the radial artery. From directional pulses one can determine whether an organ is expressing its intrinsic function or whether there is interference to that expression.

Probing pulses are the other subset of dynamic pulses and involve varying the depth of an individual finger at an individual position (cun, guan or chi) in order to obtain a reading.

Static pulses are not dynamic pulses but they are required in comprehensive pulse taking. They require no movement of the finger once the depth of interest has been reached. They include many of the famous textures of the pulse (slow, rapid, slippery, tight, thin, etc.).

POSITIONING THE BODY FOR ACCURATE PULSE DIAGNOSIS

Very often, the practitioner is seated at a desk opposite the patient. If this is the case, care should be taken to ensure that the dorsal aspect of the wrist is flat to the table. If the wrist is positioned with thumb closest to the ceiling, the reading will be focused on the Yuan-Source energetic level and will give a less accurate reading of postnatal energetics reflected in the Ying and Wei levels.

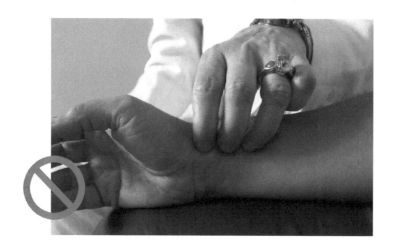

In my office I don't have a desk. I find that taking pulses while seated next to the patient on a comfortable sofa yields much more information. I sit on the right of my patients while they rest their wrists on their thighs. I take the right pulses with my left hand and then lean a little forward and take the left pulses, again with my left hand. This is a much less formal arrangement than you would have with a desk. The separation caused by a desk being placed between the patient and practitioner can result in less information being offered by the patient due to the feeling of inequality generated in that arrangement. Many practitioners, however, prefer a desk so that the wrist is level with the patient's heart.

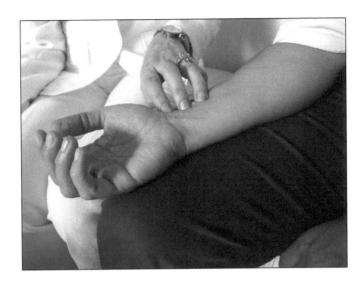

Whether behind a desk or seated next to the patient both patient and practitioner must have legs and arms uncrossed to allow Qi to flow without encumbrance.

POSITION OF THE FINGERS ON THE PULSE
To make contact with the pulse, first establish the area of the fingers that will touch the patient.

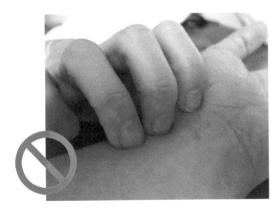

The very tips of the fingers
are less sensitive and the area presented
is too small to give
an accurate reading.

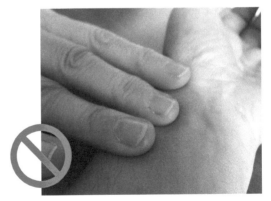

The flat part of the fingers is
too large an area to give a
concentrated reading.

The following simple exercise helps clarify the area of the practitioner's fingers that makes contact with the pulse. Bring the fingertips together to create a pyramid. The surfaces that touch are the most sensitive area of the finger.

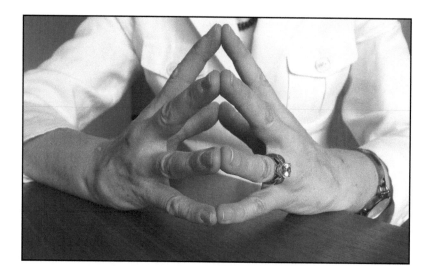

The pulses are measured at the three positions, cun, guan and chi. Each of these is one cun (one anatomical inch) apart. The inch is of course the patient's own measurement, the width of their thumb at the interphalangeal joint.

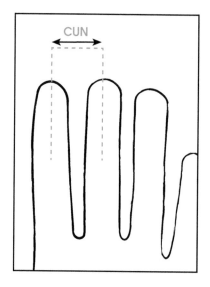

The cun position is in the area of LU-9.

The guan position is proximal to the cun by a distance of one anatomical inch.

The chi is one inch proximal to the guan.

The finger at the cun position (LU-9) can be the first to be rested on the patient, but the base of the styloid process can also be used as a starting point, making the guan position the first to be located. Place the middle finger medial to the styloid process.

If the chi position is not felt, press more deeply. If it is still not felt, move the finger at the chi position proximally in tiny increments until it appears.

Always remember to space your fingers according to the cun (measure) of the patient.
If the patient is the same height or taller than the practitioner, the practitioner's fingers will not touch each other.

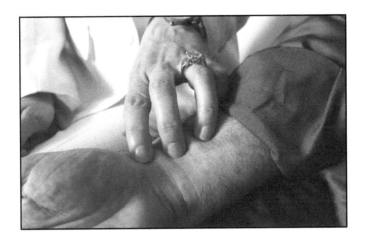

If the patient is a child, the practitioner's fingers will be very close together.

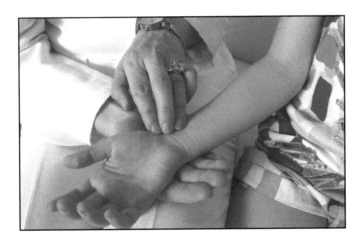

ENGENDERING PULSES IF PULSES ARE VERY WEAK OR ABSENT

Scroll One of Chapter 7 of the *Mai Jing* mentions a lost book called the *Mai Fa Zhang: Compliments of the Methods of Pulse-Taking* which talks about the union (confluent points) of the Yin and Yang organs. These points generate pulses when they cannot be found. The points where the Zang Fu meet are needled in order to generate pulses in their respective positions on the wrist.

LU-2 generates pulses in the Lung and Large Intestine positions.

LR-13 generates pulses in the Spleen and Stomach positions.

CV-4 generates pulses in the Kidney positions.

The point which is 3 fen (three tenths of a cun) below CV-15 engenders the pulse in the Heart and Small Intestine position. (Sometimes this is mistakenly translated as Du-24.) The point Bao Men which is 3 cun lateral to CV-12 generates pulses in the Liver and Gallbladder position.

Needle the appropriate point and see if that pulse emerges. You wouldn't do all of them because treatment of more than three channels is forbidden in acupuncture since it makes the Qi chaotic. Select points for needling to engender pulse based on where you wish to inquire.

Since the Lungs create the pulse in the first place and they move Blood, pulses can be engendered using the following treatment which originates in the Lung Primary Channel and ends at LU-9, the influential point that, according to the *Mai Jing*, affects all channels: CV-12, ST-25, CV-17, LU-1, LU-9.

FREQUENTLY ASKED QUESTIONS

1. *I can't find any pulses at all.*

    Move around a little. Start with the guan position and move about 2 fen (two-tenths of a cun) medial, lateral, distal and proximal. If a pulse is still not found, move more. If still not found, put the patient on the table and perform the pulse engendering treatment mentioned above.

2. *I cannot locate pulses at all in the radial artery but I do find them in the ulnar artery.*

    In rare cases, this can be so. I have even seen pulses only presenting on the dorsal aspect of the wrist.

3. *Does it really matter if the wrist is turned on its side?*

    If the thumb is facing upwards and the little finger is resting on the table, the pulses found will bring Yuan-Source level findings.

4. *I feel that when I put my finger at the styloid process all I feel is bone.*

    Move your finger slightly medially until you feel a pulse.

5. *I found two pulses in one position, slightly separate from each other. What does it mean?*

    When you have two pulses in one position, either the body has double the strength in relationship to that position or you have found a rare manifestation of a Luo pulse.

CHAPTER 2

THE NINE SPACES, THE FIVE PARAMETERS AND THE MANY PULSE TEXTURES

THE NINE SPACES

The term "Nine Spaces" refers to the three dimensional three-by-three grid in which the pulses are felt.

The three spaces in the Superficial row reflect Wei-Defensive Qi.

The three spaces in the moderate row reflect Ying-Nutritive Qi.

The three spaces in the deep row reflect Yuan-Constitutional Qi.

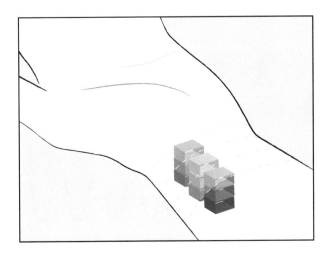 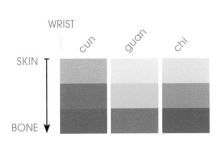

Taking pulses is like going fishing. You contact the pulse with your fingers at the nine spaces (get into your boat) and then concentrate your mind on the Five Parameters (throw out your net) and reel in the information with your mind. Then you examine and process what you have in your catch.

THE FIVE PARAMETERS

The Five Parameters of the pulse are measures of Yin and Yang. They are:

    A. Height (also known as Depth)

    B. Width

    C. Length

    D. Tempo (also known as Speed or Rate)

    E. Texture (also known as Quality or Image)

HEIGHT

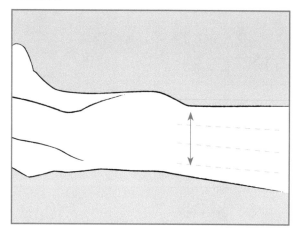

Height reflects the degree to
which Yang Qi is available and whether it is
moving up and out toward the surface.

WIDTH

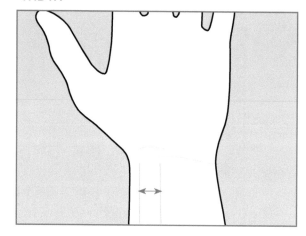

Width reflects the volume
of each of the humors.

LENGTH

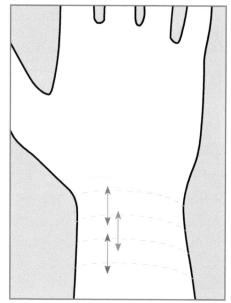

Length reflects the interplay of Yin and Yang. Qi
keeps Yin in place.

Length reflects organ strength, whether organs
are communicating with each other, whether
a disease is chronic or acute, and whether an
organ has exceeded its limits.

TEMPO

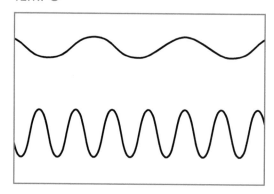

Slow (Cold)

Rapid (Heat)

TEXTURE

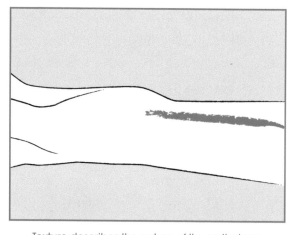

Texture describes the nature of the pathology.

HEIGHT (DEPTH)

Height (Depth) is a measure of Yang Qi. It is the Yang axis of the pulse.

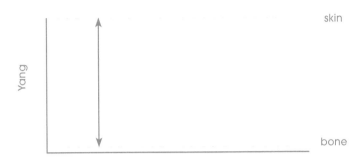

The Height of the pulse tells us how much and how well Yang Qi is moving. It reflects the vitality of Yang Qi. We are particularly interested in the capacity of Yang Qi to move pathology out to the surface for expulsion. Conversely, if there are insufficient resources to expel pathology, the height of the pulse is also a measure of the capacity of Yang Qi to bring the pathology to the Yuan level to hold it in a state of latency. The higher the Yang rises in the pulse the more it is capable of managing expulsion and latency.

The two extremes of height or depth in the pulse are:
1. The Floating pulse in which Yang is coming up to the Wei level. (In the Kidney position, this indicates a condition known as Floating Yang or Yang Escaping.)
2. The Empty pulse which indicates insufficient Yang; there is not enough Yang even to move the Qi in the pulse. This condition is known as Yang Deficiency.

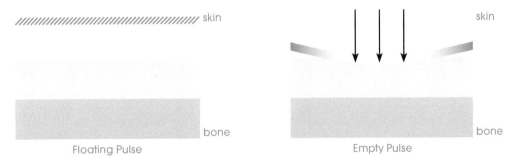

Classically, Height is said to be measured in beans. The amount of pressure you need to apply for the pulse to yield the required information is measured in the imagined weight of mung beans. This is described in Chapter 5 of the *Mai Jing* and is figurative, of course. What really matters is the distance your finger travels relative to the total depth of the pulse. The amount of pressure required to press into the bone, occluding the flow of blood in the radial artery, is said to be 15 beans. That is a standard applied to all people, so 15 beans on one person's wrist could be several times the pressure needed on another person's.

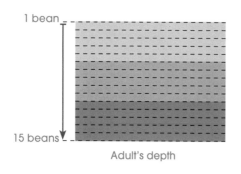

Adult's depth

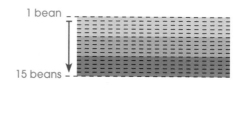

Child's depth

Divisions of the Depth of the pulse can be viewed many ways. Each of the pulses, the cun, guan and chi positions, is read at three depths: superficial, moderate and deep. Each of these depths can represent a type of Qi, a commodity, a region, an organ, or a channel. By switching lenses as we take the pulses we select what we are examining.

    1. The type of Qi (Wei, Ying and Yuan Qi).
    2. The Jin-Thin Fluids, Blood, Ye-Thick Fluids and Jing.
    3. The three Jiao's.
    4. The organs.
    5. The entire channel system.

1. DEPTH AND ITS RELATIONSHIP TO WEI, YING AND YUAN QI

WEI-defensive Qi Level	The weight of 3 beans gives a reading of the Superficial (Wei-defensive) level Wei Qi circulates in the Superficial anatomy and the Sinew and Primary Channels
YING-nutritive Qi Level	The weight of 9 beans gives a reading of the moderate (Ying-nutritive) level Ying Qi circulates in the Blood, Fluids and Primary Channels
YUAN-constitutional Qi Level	The weight of 12 beans gives a reading of the deep (Yuan-constitutional) level The weight of 15 beans gives a reading of the Hidden level. Yuan Qi circulates in the Curious Organs and the Eight Extraordinary Channels

Note: In the presence of pathology, Wei Qi circulates in the Divergent Channels and Ying Qi circulates in the Luo Channels.

This table shows the same information in more detail.

	Pressure Applied to the pulse measured in beans	Commodity Measured
SUPERFICIAL	1 to 3	The movement of Wei Qi in the Yang Sinews. The level of the Cou Li, the skin, hair and sinews (the muscles, tendons and ligaments).
SUPERFICIAL	3 to 6	The movement of Wei Qi in the Yin Sinews. The Yin Sinews control the movement of Wei Qi in the smooth muscle: the gut, heart, uterus, blood vessels, etc.
MODERATE	6 to 9	Six beans is the point at which the connection between interior and exterior is felt. The balance of Wei Qi and Ying Qi is felt. Here we see how effectively Ying Qi is converting to Wei Qi. This is where immunity is supported by digestion. The Luo Channels are also felt here.
MODERATE	9 to 11	The complement of Ying Qi: Blood and Fluids. The level of the Primary Channels. At the very bottom of this level, at around 11 beans, we find the Yang organs and the connection between the interior and the Constitution.
DEEP	12	Yin organs and their interface with Yuan Qi. The flesh which includes the deep connective tissue, the deep nerves and the fascia around the organs. At 12 beans we see the cusp of the internal and external pathways of the Primary Channels, the turning point as the internal pathways go to the organs.
HIDDEN	15	Yuan Qi. The level of Jing and the Bone. The Eight Extraordinary Channels, the Divergent Channels and the Curious Organs are felt here.

2. DEPTH AND ITS RELATIONSHIP TO JIN-THIN FLUIDS, BLOOD, YE-THICK FLUIDS AND JING

skin

	Jin-Thin Fluids	Jin-Thin Fluids circulate to the skin and the sensory orifices.
	Blood	Blood circulates in the Channels.
	Ye-Thick Fluids and Jing	Ye-Thick Fluids circulate in the Curious Organs and the Zang Fu.

bone

3. DEPTH AND ITS RELATIONSHIP TO THE THREE JIAO'S

Sometimes this is spread out; the superficial level of the cun reflects the area above the diaphragm, the moderate level of the guan reflects the area between the diaphragm and Dai Mai and the chi reflects the region below Dai Mai.

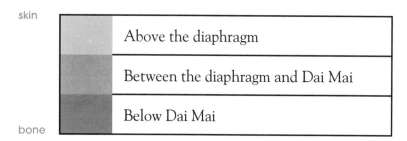

4. DEPTH AND ITS RELATIONSHIP TO THE ORGANS

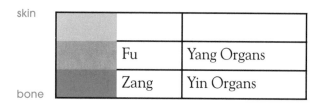

5. DEPTH AND ITS RELATIONSHIP TO THE CHANNELS

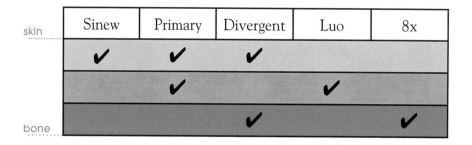

The fourth and fifth aspects of depth are often taught as a unit:

	Yang Sinew Channel
	Yang Primary Channel
	Yin Sinew Channel
	Yin Primary Channel
	Yang Organ
	Yin Organ

16

This information is important because if there is pathology in the channel but not in the organ, the prognosis is much better. Pathology detected at the organ level is serious.

If there is a pathological pulse in the Wei level and/or Ying levels, the pathology is only related to the channels. The pathology could possibly be an expression of the Zang Fu, but it is not accurate to call it an imbalance of the Zang Fu unless a pathological pulse is also found at the deep level. Keep in mind that the Yang organs are Yang expressions of the Yin organs; part of their function is to carry pathology away from their Yin-partnered organs. Pathology of the Yang organs may not be serious. However, pathology of the Yin organs is indeed serious.

RIGHT WRIST ORGANS AND CHANNELS

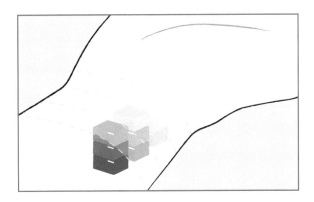

	Right cun superficial	Large Intestine Channel
	Right cun moderate	Lung Channel
		Large Intestine Organ
	Right cun deep	Lung Organ
	Right guan superficial	Stomach Channel
	Right guan moderate	Spleen Channel
		Stomach Organ
	Right guan deep	Spleen Organ
	Right chi superficial	Triple Heater Channel
	Right chi moderate	Pathology of the Pericardium and Triple Heater
	Right chi deep	Kidney Yang Pathology of TH emerges from here. (See page 195).

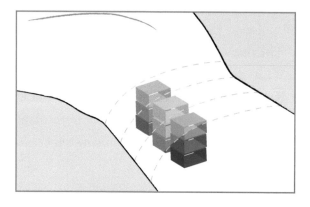

	Left cun superficial	Small Intestine Channel
	Left cun moderate	Heart Channel
		Small Intestine Organ
	Left cun deep	Heart organ
	Left guan superficial	Gallbladder Channel
	Left guan moderate	Liver Channel
		Gallbladder Organ
	Left guan deep	Liver organ
	Left chi superficial	Bladder Channel
	Left chi moderate	Kidney Channel
		Bladder Organ
	Left chi deep	Kidney Organ and Kidney Yin

SIMPLIFIED ORGAN POSITIONS

Very often this information is simplified back to a historically early form as shown here. In early pulse reading, only the Yin organs were given positions.

Right	Left
Lung	Heart
Spleen	Liver
Kidney Yang	Kidney Yin

SEASONAL AND DIURNAL INFLUENCES ON PULSE HEIGHT

There are natural rhythms in the pulses that coincide with daily and annual cycles. The pulses will tend to be higher in the wrist in spring and summer as the body resonates with the increase in Yang Qi, then deeper in the winter with the waning of Yang Qi.

The cun pulse should be higher in the morning than in the evening, as Yang Qi is prominent during the Yang period of the day, that is, the period between sunrise and the midpoint of sunrise and sunset. If the patient has called upon Yang Qi by, for example, going to the gym that morning, the pulses will tend to be yet higher.

The cun pulse should not float at all during sleep. If you come in to check pulses and the patient is asleep it would be normal to find that the pulses are deeper than when you started.

PULSES DURING MENSTRUATION

The Lung pulse gives you the status of menstruation. Diagnosis of the Lung pulse is the key to determining fertility issues.

1. During menstruation, the Lung pulse is floating because Blood is flowing out. Wei Qi is moving Blood in the uterus. Wei Qi is controlled by the Lungs.
2. As menstruation stops each month, the Lung pulse becomes floating and tight. The body is restraining Wei Qi to stop the menses.
3. At ovulation, mid-cycle, the Lung pulse is strongest at the moderate level as the Lungs begin to move Blood to the uterus. If the Lungs are not found at the moderate level or if the moderate level is thin at ovulation, either there is a Blood deficiency or there is a real or apparent Lung Qi deficiency potentially interfering with fertility. Determine the origin of the Lung Qi deficiency in cases of infertility.
4. Just prior to menses, the Lung pulse is found to be focused on the deep level as the Lungs move Blood at the level of Jing.

PSYCHOLOGICAL AND PHYSIOLOGICAL FACTORS AFFECTING PULSE DEPTH

Several factors alter the depth the pulse can rise in the wrist. Pulse reading should be calibrated to allow for these factors if you think the pulses are affected in these ways.

1. Depression
2. Privacy
3. Secrecy
4. Trauma
5. Cold
6. Damp

1. Depression can be the result of the failure of Yang Qi to move adequately, but it can also be the cause itself. Yang Qi is not able to reach its potential height if the mind has placed restrictions on the free expression of one's life force. A depressed mind seeks to minimize engagement with the outside world, causing the pulses to retreat and withdrawing vitality from the exterior.

2. Deeply private people often present with deep pulses. This is simply a result of the tendency to retract, to close in, to suppress their personality.

3. Patients may bury a pathology deep within because they may not be prepared to accept it or to share it with others at that time.

4. A history of trauma and the accompanying lack of confidence in humanity or in life can yield a feeling of protective retreat in the pulses.

5. As Cold has a constrictive nature, if the patient has internal Cold, the pulses can retract and appear deeper in the wrist. This can be simple to diagnose as the pulses will also be Tight and perhaps Slow.

6. As Damp has a heavy nature, the pulses can be covered by a layer of Dampness that makes them appear deeper in the wrist. This can be simple to diagnose as the pulses will also be Slippery.

Determining the presence of these factors is done either intuitively, or by asking the patient about the energy levels you are finding in the pulses and ensuring the Yang Qi is in fact in retreat. If the pulses all appear to be set low in the wrist but the patient has no reason to feel deficient in Yang Qi, it's likely they are affected by one of the factors listed above.

In any of these cases, the entire grid can be set down lower in the wrist. The pulse depth can be further complicated by the appearance of a thick layer of damp flesh obscuring the top of the grid. This layer is often a manifestation of protection created for the psyche.

GENERALIZED DEPTHS

The cun pulse should be felt most prominently at the superficial level because it indicates that Wei Qi is able to move to the exterior. The guan is most prominent at the moderate level because it indicates Ying Qi is being produced in the Middle Jiao. The chi pulse should be felt entirely at the deep level as Jing is precious and conserved in the Kidneys.

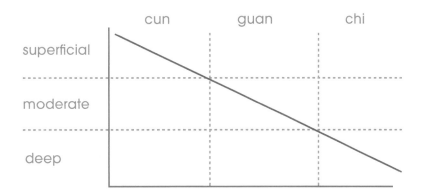

WIDTH

Width enables the practitioner to measure Yin (substance or mediumship). It is the Yin axis of the pulse.

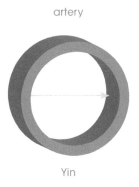

artery

Yin

The width of the pulse is provided by mediumship. In Daoist medicine it is considered hubris to determine that a pulse is too small or too big. Therefore the assessment of adequacy is made based on what you feel the pulse wants to do. Does it feel as though it wants to become bigger? Then it's thin. A Wide (Big) pulse is uncommon today because as a culture we don't cultivate our capacity to produce Yin.

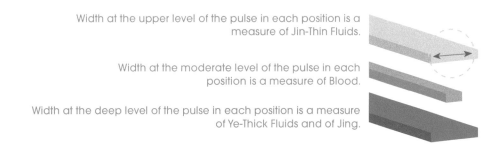

Width at the upper level of the pulse in each position is a measure of Jin-Thin Fluids.

Width at the moderate level of the pulse in each position is a measure of Blood.

Width at the deep level of the pulse in each position is a measure of Ye-Thick Fluids and of Jing.

The width of the pulse can differ in each of the three levels at the same time. These widths are examples, only.

LENGTH

Length is a measure of both Yin and Yang, including pathology related to Yin and Yang. Yang puts the pulse where it is and Yin anchors it there. The determination of whether a Long pulse refers primarily to Yin or Yang is made by analyzing other accompanying qualities in the pulses.

A Long pulse stretches beyond its position in either direction. This can be slight, where a pulse stretches slightly distally or proximally, or extreme where all three pulses are completely joined together to form one very long pulse. The extremely Long pulse occupies all three positions and indicates that there is an overflow of energy or mediumship and that the body is using the ditches (the Eight Extraordinary Channels) to absorb the excess.

Long pulses indicate either that the body is exceeding its limits or that you are feeling two organs communicating with each other. A pulse might be Long because there is too much Blood or too much Yin in the form of Dampness. Or there may be too much Qi focused on moving that medium, causing the pulse to spread. If there is much too much Qi focused on a medium, the pulse can eventually scatter. There could also be too much Wind causing the pulse to be Long. A Long pulse can also indicate Exuberant Yang.

A Short pulse indicates you either do not have enough Qi to allow the pulse to spread itself throughout its own position or not enough mediumship to fill that position. A Short pulse indicates the Yin is being contained or restrained.

The extremely Short pulse indicates insufficient Qi, insufficient mediumship or both. A short pulse can also apply to the set of three positions as a whole, when the pulse is only detected in one position or two adjacent positions.

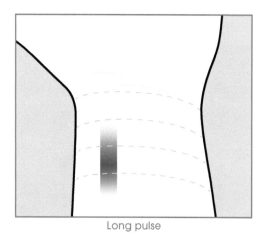

Long pulse

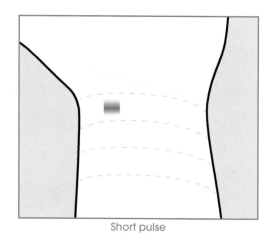

Short pulse

Tempo, the rate of the pulse, is also a measure of Yin and Yang. The rate indicates how well Qi is moving in the body. The *Mai Jing* says that every inhalation creates two heart beats during which the Qi moves three cun. Every exhalation moves Qi another three cun and creates another two beats. So a full breath has four beats and moves the Qi six cun. The rate of this movement is said to be normal when there are four pulse beats per breath.

Classically, the rate of the patient's pulse was measured against the breath of the practitioner because practitioners were considered to be at a high standard of cultivation. These days, however, as we practitioners are perhaps not adequately cultivating ourselves, the pulse rate is measured against the patient's own breath. (See counting method, page 24.) Interestingly, the word Rapid also translates as arithmetic, implying that one should count the pulses against the breath.

The clock is immaterial and not used at all. It can hinder the diagnosis. The rate must be read as a component within the individual's system, not measured by an artificial or external standard. We are interested in the relationship between the breath and the pulse in the individual.

Some positions can naturally be slightly more rapid than others. The cun is more likely to be slightly rapid than the chi position because the Qi examined in the cun is more lively than that in the chi.

Heat and Cold must be thought about in conjunction with their relationship to the Zang Fu. A Rapid pulse indicates a Yang factor is present (Heat or Heat aggravated by Wind). Yang factors cause excess movement in the pulse. Since the Fu organs express Yang Qi, a Rapid pulse is likely referring to the Fu organ of that position. Since Cold will accumulate in a Zang organ more frequently than in a Fu organ, a Slow pulse in a given position generally indicates that Cold has gone to the Zang organ of that position. It is good practice to determine first whether the Fu or the Zang organ of that position is affected and then turn the attention to Heat and Cold. Even if you were to find Heat in a Zang organ, you would have to clear Heat from the Fu pair of that organ because a key function of the Fu organs is the expression and clearing of Heat from the Zang organs. By focusing on the Fu organs, you are focusing on clearing the Heat.

A Slow or hesitant pulse indicates a Yin factor is present (Cold or Damp). The Yin factor is impeding the movement of the pulse. By its nature Cold is very restrictive and brings things into the deeper level. The disease can move deeper, into the Zang organ, so the Zang organ should be on your mind. The central tenet of the classical tradition is to anticipate the transmission of disease and to treat preventatively, arresting the progression of disease. Knowing the current location of the Cold enables us to deduce the path it might take and prevent that progression. Breaking up the Cold before it can go into that deeper level is the action required for healing.

Tempo can vary not only from one pulse position to another, but also from one depth to another within the same pulse position. Therefore the pulse rate at each of the positions is measured, as is the rate at each of the three depths. This sounds like a tall order, but it is done quite swiftly. You will notice immediately if the pulse is faster or slower as you shift your attention. The pulse rate can differ markedly in each position. It is possible to find the Kidneys at four beats per breath and the Spleen at seven beats per breath. One time I found the Lungs at three beats per breath and the Liver concurrently at 14 beats per breath. These discrepancies occur as the blood vibrates differently in the different positions, reflecting the Qi of the individual organs. These variations enable the practitioner to accurately locate the Heat or Cold.

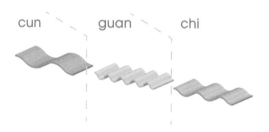

The tempo can be different in each position at the same time.

MEASURING PULSE TEMPO

Tempo, the measure of the pulse on the continuum from slow to rapid is determined by counting the number of beats per patient breath. Often I am asked how this can be done without staring directly at a patient impolitely. Here is the method I use:

1. Assume your pulse-taking posture.
2. Cast your gaze at a point beyond the patient, to one side, as though you are looking perhaps at the floor, a few feet behind them.
3. Keeping your eyes focused on that point, notice the movements of the patient's chest.
4. If they have loose clothing on, notice the top of the shoulder, without looking at it directly.
5. Identify the point of highest expansion of the chest, the peak of the breath.
6. Count the number 1 at the highest point of the next breath and keep counting the pulse beats: 1, 2, 3, etc.

7. At the peak of the next breath, count the number one again and keep counting the pulse beats, 1, 2, 3, etc.

8. At the peak of the next breath, count one again and keep counting, 1, 2, 3, etc.

9. Do this perhaps three times and see what number you reach each time. The number can differ slightly as no person breathes at a consistent rate.

10. The average rate is considered the rate of the patient's pulse.

TEXTURE

The textures of the pulses fall generally into two categories: excess or deficient. Deficient pulses include the textures Empty, Weak, Soft, Frail, Minute. Excess textures reflect the presence of accumulations and include Full, Leathery, Firm, Wiry, Tight. Texture is determined in the pulses by applying pressure to and/or releasing pressure from the radial artery and sensing subtle behaviors and qualities in the pulse. When analyzing textures, first feel whether the pulse is strong or weak. Then examine the texture. Textures are listed below in the order in which I have found it easiest to discuss them.

TEXTURES OF THE PULSE

1. Weak, Insufficient	13. Long	26. Floating
1A. Frail, Minute	14. Slippery	26A. Flooding, Surging
2. Exuberant, Full	15. Beady	26B. Hollow, Scallion
3. Rapid	16. Not-Rested	27. Soft
4. Slow	17. Empty	28. Urgent
5. Tight	18. Faint, Frail	29. Hasty
6. Wiry, Bowstring	19. Scattered	30. Knotted
7. Thin, Small	20. Leathery, Taut	31. Intermittent
8. Choppy	21. Firm	
9. Rough	22. Hidden	
10. Narrow, Fine	23. Moving, Vibrating	
11. Big, Wide	24. Normal	
12. Short	25. Superficial	

1. WEAK, INSUFFICIENT

A Weak pulse indicates insufficient activity in that position. The pulse falls well short of feeling vital. The Weak pulse doesn't have much definition. It results from a deficiency of Qi.

A Weak pulse can result after many other qualities have been experienced; it can be the Yin result of too much Yang having been accumulated. For example, a Wiry pulse which formed

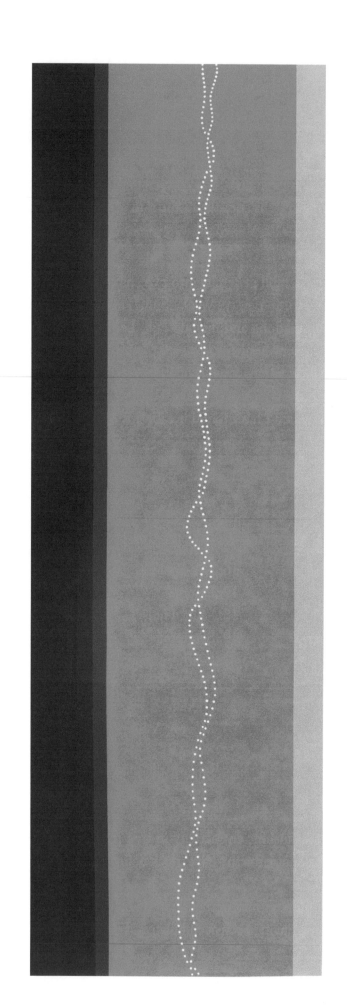

The Weak Pulse

Pulses, pathological or not, can be beautiful since they are microcosms of humanity. Strength and hope
are restored through the insights gained during pulse-taking.

due to long-term anger can become so Wiry and consume so much energy that the pulse reaches a point where it cannot sustain the wiry quality and must transform. It flips, leaving it Weak. At that point, the anger transmutes into depression. Suddenly as a result you have Weak pulses with hints that it was once Wiry; it may be Weak with a hint of tightness.

The term Weak can describe a lack of strength at the deep level, especially in the Kidneys as they support the Spleen. Weak can also be used as a relative term to indicate strength when compared with adjacent pulses. When a moderate level pulse disappears as it is pressed to the Yuan level, it can be considered Weak.

Feels like: The Weak pulse gives you the feeling of lack of confidence in that organ or in the fluids of that position.

1A. FRAIL OR MINUTE

The Frail or Minute pulse is a subset of the Weak pulse. It feels almost wispy, indicating great Weakness. It is even weaker than the Weak pulse.

Feels like: When pressure is increased, the Frail or Minute pulse disappears..

2. EXUBERANT, FULL

These pulses have strength and liveliness and are the opposite of Weak. They illustrate that Yang Qi is plentiful. Healthy children have Exuberant pulses. Sometimes the word Full is used to indicate a lot of sensation in the pulse implying excess Yang. Classically these pulses were sometimes called Big or Wide. Today we don't use these terms much; we simply use the term Full. The term Big means the vessel is very dilated, an excessive version of Full.

Feels like: Full or Exuberant pulses feel round and relaxed, coming up to meet your finger with an abundance of Qi. These pulses give you confidence that there is adequate mediumship and that the associated organs are strong.

3. RAPID

A Rapid pulse indicates that the movement of Qi is being increased by a Yang factor: Heat, or Wind with Heat. A Rapid pulse has more than four beats per breath. Five beats per breath could be called slightly Rapid, seven beats would be very Rapid. The more Rapid the pulse, the more heat there is trapped in that organ or in the mediumship of that position. See also tempo, page 23.

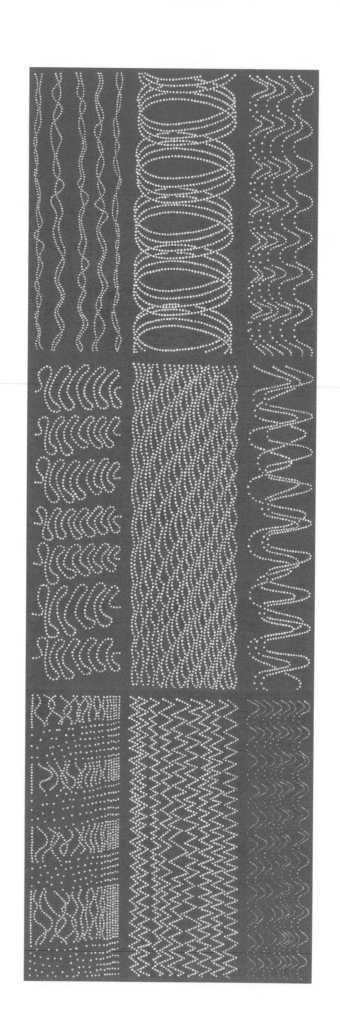

The Rapid Pulse

It's important to remember that a pulse can be Rapid in any or many locations in the pulse, in the cun, guan, chi positions and at the Wei, Ying and Yuan levels. Here we see a sampler of variations on the Rapid pulse. From left to right and from Wei to Yuan levels, the pulse is rapid and: superficial, flooding, weak, tight, slippery (center), choppy, thin, moving and beginning to float.

Feels like: Even before counting the rate, the Rapid pulse has at least some degree of urgency about it.

4. SLOW

A Slow pulse indicates that the movement of Qi is being impeded by a Yin factor: Cold or Damp. A Slow pulse is defined as fewer than four beats per breath. (The Slowest pulse I have felt is just over one beat per breath in a man who grew up in Moscow during the 1930s without winter shoes.)

5. TIGHT

Perhaps the most misunderstood pulse in Chinese medicine, the Tight pulse is of great importance. Treatment to directly release Tight pulses can result in worsening a condition. Tight pulses are usually not an indicator of pathology but show the body's appropriate response to pathology; the body is trying to conserve a medium (Fluids, Blood or Jing). The body is trying to minimize the consumption of these resources because it recognizes that they are deficient. For example, a woman presenting with debilitating migraines and a very Tight, Thin Liver pulse has a severe Blood deficiency to which the Liver is responding by trying to restrict the flow of Blood. She is in need of strong nourishment of Blood. The Tightness in the pulse must be left alone so as not to disrupt her body's conservation of Blood. To release the Tightness is to fail to respect that the body is responding perfectly to the cause of the migraines. Releasing the Tightness does not help her body conserve the Blood she presently has, or the Blood to be built through treatment. When the Blood is built back, the Tightness in the pulse can simply disappear, along with the migraines.

Feels like: The Tight pulse feels as though pressure is being applied along the sides of the radial artery. This pressure is constricting the vessel, pushing inward. If you roll your finger laterally, you'll find there is a distinct border. This verifies Tightness. A hallmark of the Tight pulse is that the pressure along the sides of the artery causes the top of the pulse to move upward with every beat. The top of the artery hits the finger with every beat at a higher level than it would otherwise.

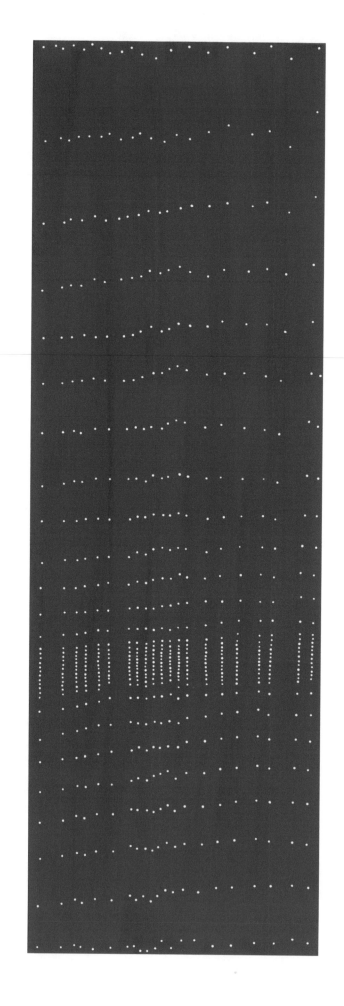

The Slow Pulse

A pulse becomes slow when it is influenced by a Yin factor, be it Cold or Damp. This is the pulse of a patient who spent his entire life in Russia, growing up without winter shoes, witnessing horrific violence, then maturing into a man of great dignity but with unspeakable pain. His pulse, which ran at about one and a half beats per breath, was informed by suppressed fear, cold, damp, and the determination to maintain meaningful connections with his family and friends.

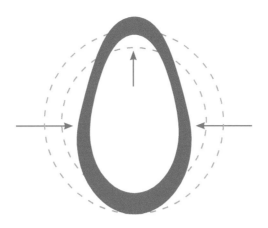

The tight pulse feels as though it is being pushed in from the sides.

A Tight pulse means the organ or the mediumship of that position is resisting movement. This stagnation can either be of Yin or Yang. For example, if there is a deficiency of Ye-Thick Fluids, the Small Intestine pulse can tighten in order to restrict Ye-Thick Fluids in an attempt to consolidate them. Or, the body might be consolidating resources in response to a pathogenic factor, preparing for a healing crisis.

The level at which the Tightness is present in the pulse indicates the mediumship the body is trying to gather. If the pulse is Tight and Floating it may be gathering Wei Qi or Jin-Thin Fluids.

If Tight at the moderate level it may be gathering Ying, or Blood. If Tight at the deep level it may be gathering Yuan Qi or Jing. A Tight pulse may seem like an excess pulse, but if you press down further, probing it, you may find a Weakness underlying the Tightness. The show of excess is the body's attempt to respond to the loss of resources. This is an appropriate or physiological response.

If a pulse is Tight pathologically, however, which is less common, it indicates stagnation. Cold is the chief cause of stagnation manifesting as Tightness in the pulse. Damp causes resistance too, but a Damp, Tight pulse is called Slippery. Tight pulses can be Slow, reflecting the Cold, or Rapid, indicating the beginning of the generation of Heat in response to Cold. Since Cold has a constrictive quality, a Tight pulse can indicate lateral, costal and flank pain. Tightness can also indicate the consumption of Yang, which results in Cold. True stagnation is present in a pulse that does not give way. If a Tight quality is found but gives way when you push beyond it, it is technically not a Tight pulse, but Leathery, Firm, or Hidden. (See page 45.) A pulse could be Tight perhaps on the surface level and then Hidden on the deep level. That would technically not be a pulse of true stagnation.

Psychologically a Tight pulse can mean resistance to change, physical hesitation, sluggishness or fatigue.

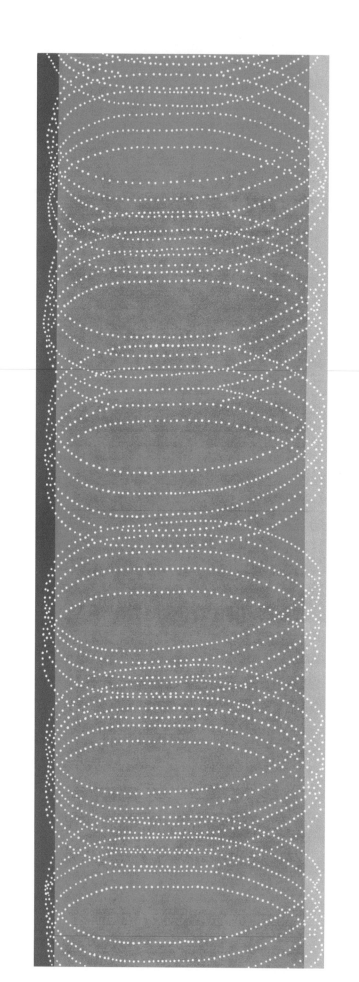

Tight Pulse

When the pulse is tight, it feels as though something is pressing in on the sides, constricting it and causing the top of the pulse to move upward, into the practitioner's finger. A tight pulse is an opportunity for the practitioner to cultivate calm while taking the pulse, coaxing the pulse into a relaxed, healing state.

Long-term Tight pulses become Rapid eventually as the Wei Qi involved in the stagnation becomes concentrated Heat. As the height increases (the Yang axis of the pulse), the width decreases (the Yin axis of the pulse). This is what is meant by the notion that Yang is always affected before Yin. For example, Qi is affected before Blood. The tightness prevents Yin moving effectively and when the Yin cannot move, a slippery quality develops.

The good news about a Tight pulse is that the patient is not Weak. You need Qi to generate the Tightness.

6. WIRY (SOMETIMES CALLED BOWSTRING)

Feels like: Wiry means that you have constriction all around the vessel, as though the radial artery is cinched or gripped by a belt along its entire circumference. A Wiry pulse stays constricted at all pressures without any hollowing or giving way. If a pulse is very Wiry, often you cannot push it down to the level below it.

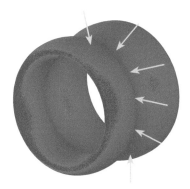

A Wiry pulse indicates long-term Qi stagnation. An extended period of Long pulses precedes the formation of Wiry pulses. Long pulses indicate the body is exceeding its limits by retaining too much Dampness, or even too much mediumship (Blood and Fluids). If this goes on long enough and is not addressed, the body can eventually try to rein in the excess to contain it, in an attempt to stop the body containing more. During that process and as a result of that process, the pulses become strangulated, Wiry. This is an example of the conversion of Yin to Yang; the body has created resistance and closure after an untenable situation reached its limits. A long-term overflow of Yin leads to the summoning of Yang to control it.

Since a Wiry pulse is a pulse of constraint, emotions are not in free flow and frustration sets in. A Wiry pulse often reveals a patient's feeling of deep constraint. There might be a feeling of being trapped or a feeling that there is no opportunity for any sense of liberation. This could also manifest as physical pain. There may be a sense of suffocation or a feeling that there is nothing to stimulate a sense of animation or action. If very Wiry, anger can transmute to violence.

If a Wiry quality perseveres, Qi is depleted to the point where the stagnation cannot be maintained and the pulses become Weak with an echo of Tightness. This is how anger transmutes into depression. Wiry pulses in the Kidney position are a sign of stagnation of the Will; depression worsens.

A Wiry pulse can also indicate a heightened attempt to secure latency of a pathogenic factor. If the Kidneys are weak, the body may stagnate Yin and bring it to the Kidneys to support latency. The Yin holds Qi to support Yang. As a result there could be Blood stasis, Phlegm stasis or Qi stasis.

A Wiry pulse can indicate an extreme deficiency of a resource and the resulting extreme Tightness as the body tries valiantly to contain what resources it does have. This can apply to deficiencies of Jing, Yin, Yang or Qi but generally the underlying deficiency is more difficult to find in very Wiry pulses because of the intensity of the stagnation.

Wiry pulses lead to Heat as the body tries to create movement to restore the flow of Qi.

If the pulse is Tight and Thin, rather than Wiry, the feeling of volume changes from level to level. A truly Wiry pulse is consistent through the levels.

7. THIN OR SMALL

A Thin pulse indicates a deficiency of mediumship. The medium that is deficient can be determined by the depth and the pulse position. For example, a Thin pulse in the moderate level of the Liver position indicates a deficiency of Blood. A Thin pulse in the deep level of the left Kidney pulse would indicate a deficiency of Jing. Classically, a Thin pulse does not describe the width felt. A Thin pulse is one in which you feel the artery not filling with mediumship sufficiently to create an outward pressure on the internal walls of the artery.

Feels like: You are aware of the blood flowing through the artery but no pressure is felt moving outward from the interior of the artery. No Qi is felt moving outward in the artery wall. A Thin pulse has the feeling that the wall wants to dilate but can't because there's not enough mediumship helping to generate a vibration.

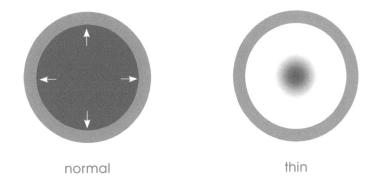

normal   thin

A thin pulse feels as though it wants to fill up, to be bigger in all directions.

8. CHOPPY

A Choppy pulse is either Thin and Tight or Thin and Wiry. It feels Choppy because the lack of mediumship causes the co-existing Tightness to constrict the pulse further, driving the top of the pulse into a point at your finger. The flow of blood is obstructed as the vessel is squeezed, stagnating the blood. The medium the body is trying to accumulate is demonstrated by the level at which the choppiness peaks. If the point of the pulse reaches up to the Wei level, the body is either trying to accumulate Wei Qi or Jin-Thin Fluids. If the point of the pulse comes up to the moderate level, the body is trying to accumulate Blood. If the point only reaches within the Yuan level, the body is trying to accumulate Ye-Thick Fluids or Jing.

Feels like: The area of your finger the pulse hits is very fine, like the point of a cleaver.

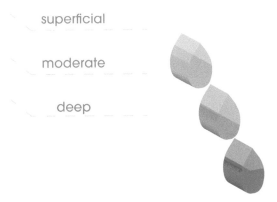

superficial

moderate

deep

The tip of a choppy pulse can be focused in any of the three levels.

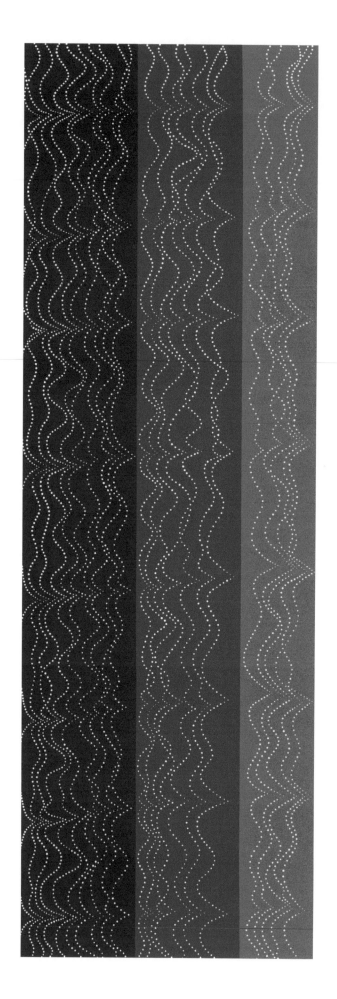

The Choppy Pulse

A Choppy pulse is either Thin and Tight or Thin and Wiry. It feels Choppy because the lack of mediumship causes the co-existing tightness to constrict the pulse further, driving the top of the pulse into a point at your finger. This pulse is a reminder to invite the patient to honor themselves: to rest, sleep early, enjoy good nourishment and relax into the feeling of being intuitively guided.

9. ROUGH

This is the same word as Choppy in Chinese but in practice the Rough pulse is a variation of the Choppy pulse. A Rough pulse is a Choppy pulse that hits many different places on the diagnosing finger, sometimes feeling as though it is approaching the finger from many different angles. This indicates that the volume of mediumship (Blood or Fluids) has decreased enough to allow Wind to enter the channel, causing instability.

Feels like: The Rough pulse feels as though a ball point pen is tapping at your finger from a different angle and landing at a slightly different spot on the finger at every strike.

10. NARROW, FINE

These pulses indicate a dearth of mediumship and Qi. Depending on the position, there is insufficient Jin-Thin Fluids, Blood, Ye-Thick Fluids, or Jing. The Thin pulse indicates a deficiency of mediumship whereas the Narrow pulse indicates that both mediumship and Qi are deficient.

Feels like: At the extreme end of the Narrow spectrum, the pulse feels like a fine thread under the finger.

11. BIG, WIDE

This reflects adequate or excess mediumship. Depending on the position and depth, there is sufficient Jin-Thin Fluids, Blood, Ye-Thick Fluids, or Jing. This pulse is seldom seen. If the pulse is very broad and Floating, there is likely a leakage of fluids; mediumship is escaping and coming to the superficial level. If leaking blood, it might be Big at the moderate level. Wide pulses can show that there may be excess Yin attempting to accommodate a deficiency. They can also indicate Blood stagnation. The term Big can mean that mediumship has overflowed.

Feels like: These pulses feel as though they make contact with a broad section of the finger.

The next two pulses describe length.

12. SHORT

A Short pulse doesn't even fill its own position. There is either insufficient mediumship to fill the position, or there is insufficient Yang Qi to hold the mediumship in place. The short quality can result from a blockage, stagnation or accumulation, preventing movement.

Feels like: The Short pulse feels as though it contacts a very Small area of the finger.

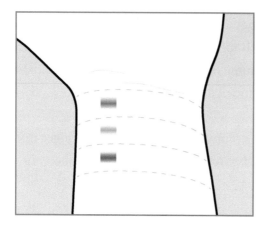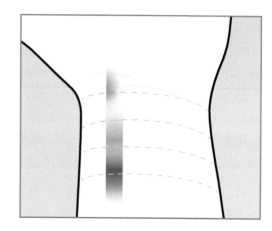

13. LONG

A Long pulse indicates a pathological excess of Yin and its interplay with Qi. It could be excess Damp, Blood or Fluids. Yin can overflow and fill up more than one position. The body has not recognized its own limits and has exceeded its capacity. For example, if there is too much Blood, you might feel that the Liver pulse and the Heart pulse are felt as one Long position as the excess Blood stored in the Liver floods up to the Heart. A Long pulse can result from pathogenic factors also, as the body tries to shift pathology from one location or one level of Qi or Fluids to another.

Long-term Long pulses eventually flip, as conversion from a Yin state to a Yang state occurs. The body creates resistance to overflow and a Wiry pulse can sometimes result. The body is tempering its own tendency to exceed its own capacity.

A person might be exceeding his or her emotional limits also. Long-term anger can lead to a Long, Wiry Liver pulse that extends beyond the parameters of the guan position to include the cun position. Over time, a Long pulse might send its excess to the ditches (the Eight Extraordinary Channels) as the limits of this aspect of the patient are exceeded. This is why the Eight Extraordinary pulses tend to be Long pulses. A long pulse can become empty or change quality as it moves to another channel.

A long or overflowing pulse can indicate something trapped where it should not be. Long towards the thumb reflects Yin being trapped on the Yang surface, perhaps as Ying is converting to Wei Qi.

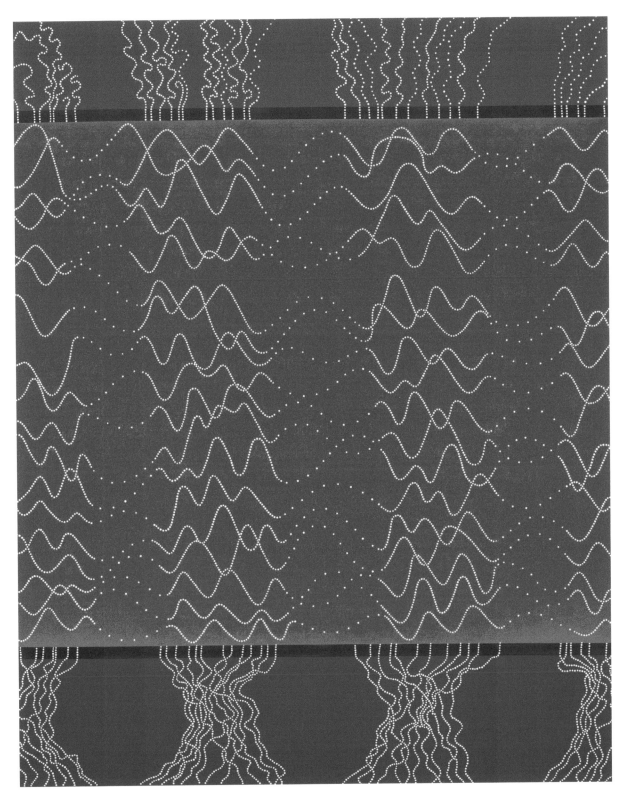

The Big Pulse

The pulse is big and joyous if the Blood is joyous. The root of all Qi (Yuan Qi) creates the postnatal arena where a dedicated sensitivity and responsiveness to the steering feelings in the belly result in true joy that is then transmitted and shared for the benefit of all.

14. SLIPPERY

The Slippery pulse indicates the presence of Dampness.

Diet is not the only cause of Dampness, of course. Over thinking weakens the Spleen, making it less able to resolve Dampness.

The word slippery also implies tightness. This is for two reasons: firstly, Dampness constricts the flow of Qi, Yin, Blood and Fluids, and secondly, areas that are deficient are tight because of a mechanism of compensation. The body is trying to retain the medium it feels is in short supply. The Slippery pulse is sometimes considered to measure equally in its lateral and vertical cross-section, giving it a "diameter". A Slippery pulse is generally Rapid because where there is Damp stagnation there is Heat, as the body uses Heat to break up the stagnation. The emergence of Slippery pulses during the early phases of digestion and during pregnancy is normal and does not need to be treated.

Feels like: The Slippery pulse has a lingering quality and goes away from your finger slowly. Li Shi Zhen describes it as being like pearls slipping under the fingers. It has no distinct border and is consonant-free. A Normal pulse begins with a firm consonant, Baah, Baah, Baah, Baah, Baah, or Daah, Daah, Daah, Daah, Daah, but a Slippery pulse begins with a vowel or an H: haah, haah, haah, or errr, errr, errr or uhhh, uhhh, uhhh. Over the years I've practiced guessing the chief culprit of the Dampness in the Spleen position. Cheese is the easiest to detect because it has a sticky heaviness to it regardless of the rate: errr errr errr. The cheese-induced Slippery pulse feels like melted thick mozarella and is very sluggish. The gluten pulse has an airiness to it, a kind of dense puffiness, and lacks depth, almost like highly processed white bread: huuh, huuh, huuh. The Slippery pulse that has sugar as the principal culprit is characterized by a flat shapelessness: aaa, aaa, aaa. The pulse doesn't rise well and feels like a wet, failed soufflé. Many people eat all three categories regularly, but detection is becoming easier as more people make the decision to cut out one or two of the three.

15. BEADY

The Beady pulse indicates long-term stagnation of Dampness or Blood resulting in Yin or Blood stasis.

Feels like: The Beady pulse feels like a small pearl, very compact, compressed and slippery. It can feel like a cyst or fibrotic tissue. As you push into it, it continues to show delineated borders.

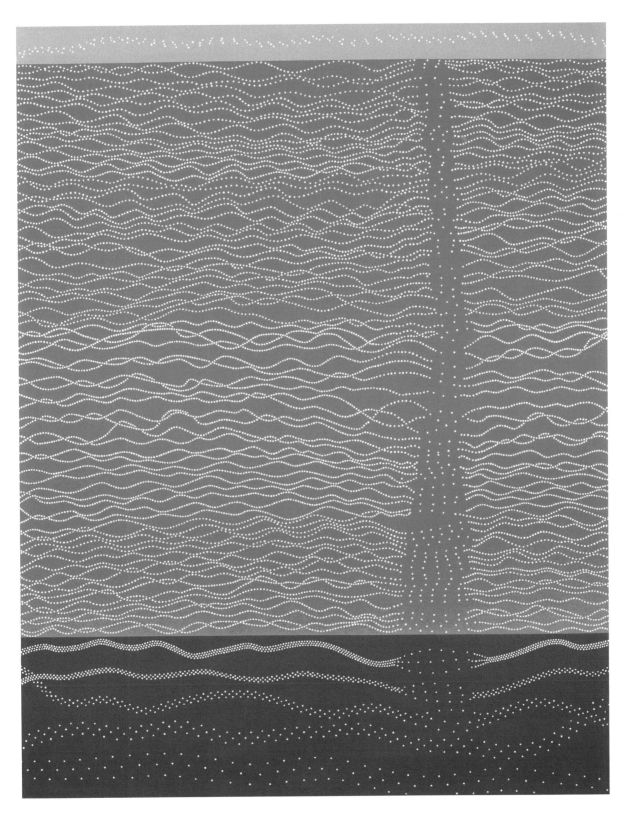

Slippery Pulse

The slippery pulse lacks definition or a consonant at the commencememt of the beat. This can be because the body is busy transforming sticky substances, but the slippery pulse is present in everyone after a meal or during pregnancy. Hence, it can be a pulse of richness and repleteness, of ripeness and relish.

16. NOT-RESTED

Usually found in the Spleen or Heart position, this pulse indicates difficulty in gathering resources or feeling grounded at home or at work. In the Heart position it can mean Wei Qi is not anchoring at night; Blood is not being restored.

Feels like: There are two manifestations of the Not-Rested pulse:
1. The pulse meets the finger at erratically varying pressures. Some beats feel stronger than others.
2. The pulse varies erratically in height, sometimes meeting the finger and sometimes not.

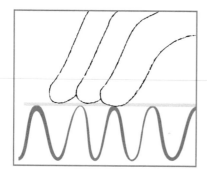 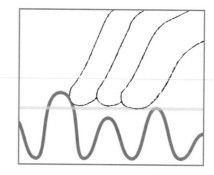

17. EMPTY

The Empty pulse indicates insufficient Yang Qi. The term Empty does not imply that there is no pulse in that position.

Feels like: After finding a pulse on any level, if you increase pressure on the pulse and find that it then disappears, you have found an empty pulse.

Comparison with Hidden: The Hidden pulse is one that appears after pressure is applied to 15 beans of pressure.

Note: If no pulse is found because something is obstructing the pulses, preventing them from emerging, a treatment is done to harmonize the pulses in order to generate them. See page 9.

HIDDEN WEAKNESS, ARMORING AND LATENCY

The next few pulses indicate the presence of hidden weakness (18, 19), armoring (20, 21) or latency (22, 23). They all involve tightness. The tightness is again due to an underlying deficiency; the body can stagnate or hold on to the Blood to conserve it, causing the pulse to become Taut or Leathery. The inadequacy of the underlying mediumship is confirmed by the presence of weakness beneath the tightness. The armoring we feel in the pulse illustrates that the body has its guard up against further depletion of mediumship. Underneath that armor is a discernible hidden weakness. The tightness involved in the following pulses therefore shows a false excess.

Latency is a term for the state of a pathogen when it is being hidden by the body so that it cannot reach the viscera. Latency occurs when the body has not been able to deal with a pathogenic factor. The body recognizes that the disease of an internal organ is the most serious of all illnesses. Using very sophisticated strategies (described by the Complement Channels), the body shifts a pathogen out of the Primary Channels to ensure the safety of the organs or, in the case of the Sinew Channels, prevents penetration of the Primary Channels altogether. In the presence of a potentially life-threatening disease the Complement Channels move the illness away from the Zang Fu, into latency (into hiding) creating a different, "slower" disease so that the viscera are preserved. The Complement Channels are present literally to preserve humanity. Once the containment of pathology is assured (once latency is achieved), symptoms fade away—the patient appears to get better and life goes back to normal. The pulses, however, do not go back to normal; they clearly show the pathogen's presence, albeit in latency.

18. FAINT/FRAIL

The Faint/Frail pulses indicate a lack of strength and width, manifesting most often in the guan position. A Faint pulse is a Weak pulse with almost no width. It feels almost wispy. A Faint pulse in the right guan position indicates that there is not enough strength in the Spleen or Stomach to produce and transport Fluids and manage and maintain Blood. In the left guan it indicates that there is not enough strength to store Blood.

Comparison with Empty: The Empty pulse disappears with pressure; the Faint is barely present to begin with.

Comparison with Weak: The Weak pulse is lacking in force but absence of width is not necessarily implied.

19. SCATTERED

The opposite of Full, the Scattered pulse demonstrates a shortage of mediumship. There is not enough mediumship to fill the channel and maintain the movement of Blood in its vessel in a streamlined way. A Floating and Weak pulse at the cun position is often called Scattered.

Feels like: A healthy pulse exhibits strength against the finger but a Scattered pulse disperses

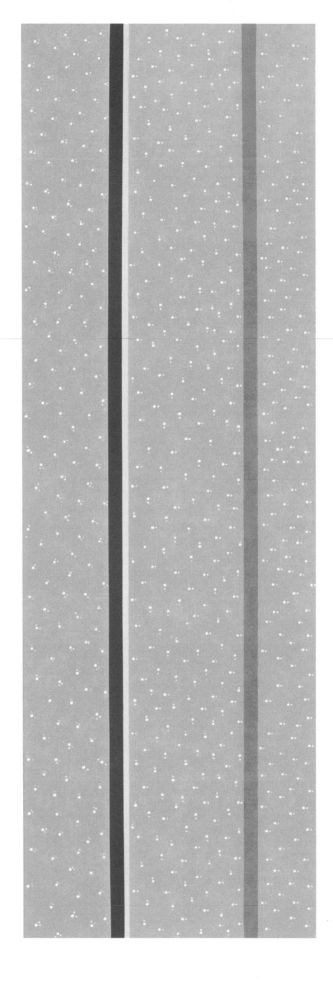

The Scattered Pulse

in many directions like fireworks. Energy is felt moving up and out. A Scattered pulse has no integrity as you lift your finger and is unable to follow the pressure applied to it while maintaining its shape. It breaks up as pressure on it is reduced.

Note: A pulse should not scatter as it hits the finger unless it is within the superficial level of the cun pulse. The Heart and Lung pulses should scatter to some degree because it is the nature of the Heart and Lungs to interact with the world.

Comparison with Soft: The term Scattered means there is no integrity as your finger is moving upward. In general, the term Soft means that there is little integrity as you are pressing downward. A pulse should not soften like cotton when pressure is applied to it.

LEATHERY, FIRM AND HIDDEN

The next three pulses, Leathery, Firm and Hidden are all subsets of the Full pulse. The level at which you find a tight banded quality is what will determine whether it is Leathery, Firm or Hidden. If it emerges as you press just a little beyond the Wei level, the pulse is Leathery. If it emerges as you press just a little beyond Ying level, the pulse is Firm. If it emerges as you release pressure after going into the bone, the pulse is Hidden.

20. LEATHERY, TAUT

A Leathery pulse is specific to examination between the superficial and moderate levels. The Leathery pulse demonstrates a leakage of Qi or the inability of Qi to move upward. It shows a significant underlying deficiency complicated by a great effort to appear strong. Leathery pulses can also mean that there is some type of stagnation at either the Blood (moderate) level or in the Yuan (deep) level preventing the patient from having full resolution of their imbalance. The origin, of course, will be some kind of Qi and/or Blood stagnation responding to the deficiency of a medium, but the visual appearance of the patient will often not betray that deficiency. You won't know it until you examine the pulse and find that belying the appearance of the patient is a significant deficiency. I think of this as being like a physical stoicism.

Feels like: The Leathery pulse has three stages of sensation as you increase pressure: Fullness, then resistance, then emptiness.

Stage 1. Fullness: At first the Leathery pulse is either Floating and Tight or feels full under the finger. However this fullness is a false one. That fullness that you felt initially was present only to provide for the resistance.

Stage 2. Resistance: When you press down on a Leathery pulse between the superficial and moderate levels, it becomes apparent that there is something in the central area of the pulse (not at the sides of the pulse) blocking your finger's journey into the pulse. You feel

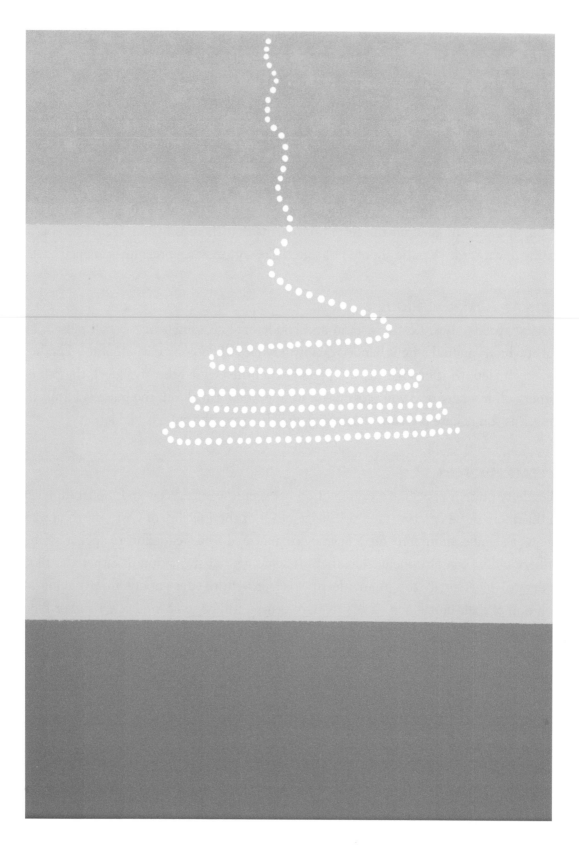

The Leathery Pulse

something resisting you in the superficial level, something trying to prevent you from going into the moderate level. Upon pressure the pulse becomes long, like a flat band under your finger at the moderate level.

Stage 3. Emptiness: When you press beyond the band, an emptiness is revealed and the pulse disappears. What appeared to be an excess was not a true excess but an armoring, a guarding of the remaining complement of the resource that was lost or not built. The person does not have the integrity to build the resource back, but they do have the strength to attempt to guard or armor their present weakness, creating a Leathery quality in the pulse.

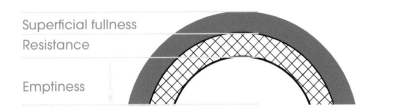 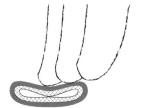

Superficial fullness

Resistance

Emptiness

Three Stages of Leathery Pulse

Comparison with Tight and Wiry: A Leathery pulse has resistance at the center of the vessel. A Tight pulse has resistance at the sides of the vessel. A Wiry pulse has resistance in the circumference of the vessel.

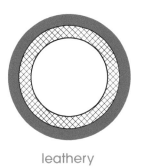 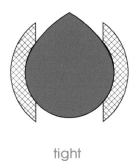 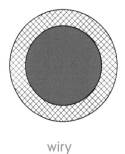

leathery   tight   wiry

Comparison with Hollow: Leathery should not be confused with Hollow. Hollow implies that as you push down, it feels very vulnerable underneath. There is no band.

Comparison with Long: The Long pulse shows that there is a weakness in the ascension of energy and that the Qi is leaking back down away from the Upper Jiao. In the Lung position, for example, the Long pulse indicates breathing problems; the Qi is not going up and out. The Long pulse shows that the body is trying to hold onto Qi because Qi and/or Blood have been lost or are collapsing.

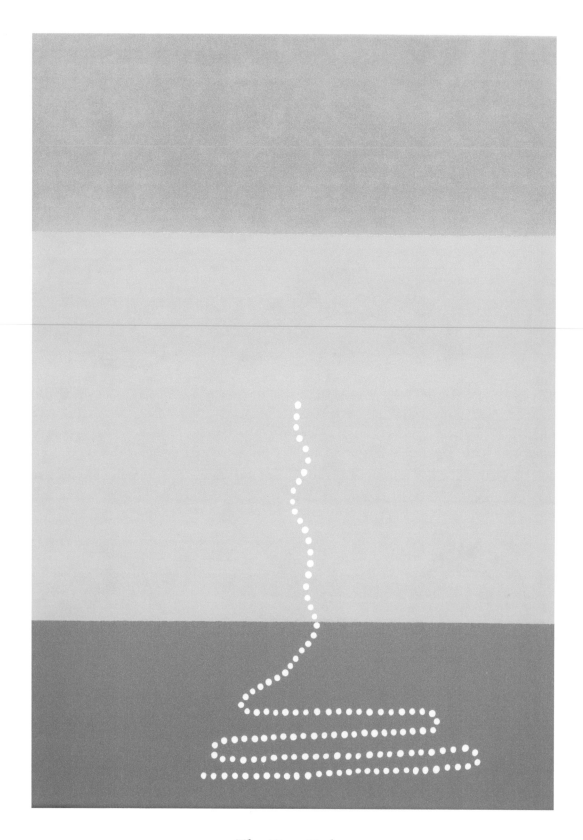

The Firm Pulse

21. FIRM

The Firm pulse is one that becomes Long when you push down from the moderate level into the deep level. This indicates leakage of Blood or Ying. It is Firm because the mediumship or its Qi is leaking out and the body is trying to hold on to it.

Feels like: When you press from the moderate level and are about to go to the deep level you feel resistance to your finger proceeding. As you keep pressing, a wide taut band appears; this is the key characteristic of the Firm pulse. Pressing beyond that band reveals an emptiness. The pulse disappears. What appeared to be an excess was in fact an armoring, a guarding of the remaining complement of the resource that had been lost.

Comparison with Leathery: Both the Firm and Leathery pulses have the same feeling about them. They are differentiated by the depth at which the resistance (the leatheriness or firmness) is felt. A Floating and Full banded pulse which empties upon pressure is a Leathery pulse. A moderate and Full banded pulse that empties upon pressure is a Firm pulse.

22. HIDDEN

The Hidden pulse (Fu Mai) is one that only reveals itself after the bone has been palpated. It indicates that there is pathology latent in the constitutional level. It is referred to as Hidden because it was there all the time but unrevealed until the Yuan level was stimulated. The Hidden pulse is also called the Stone pulse in the *Nan Jing*.

Feels like: As you palpate the pulse you might feel some indication of various things on the way but there is little felt in the Yuan level of the pulse. Press all the way into the bone (15 beans of pressure). When you release back up to 14 beans of pressure, a pulse does clearly appear in the Yuan level. The Hidden pulse indicates Eight Extraordinary or Divergent Channel pathology. See chapter 5.

15 beans of pressure   14 beans of pressure

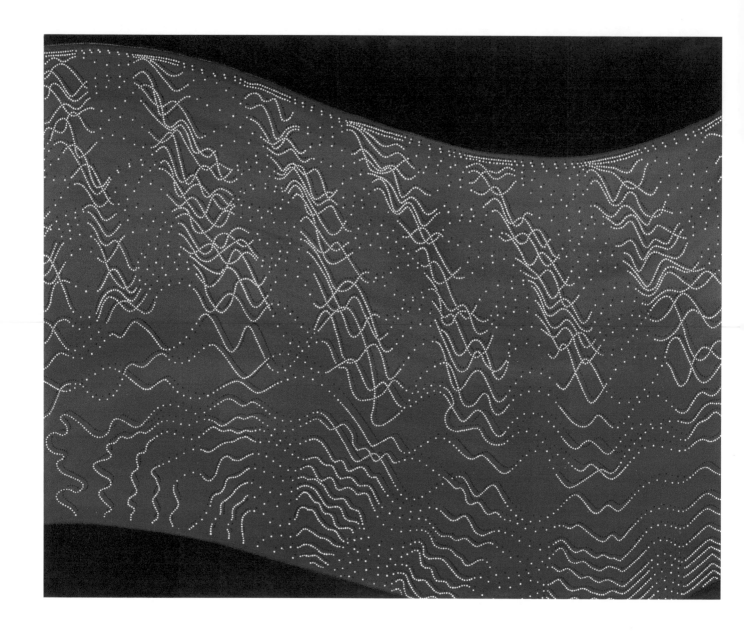

The Moving Pulse

This painting describes the energetic impact of the entry of a pathogen. In Chinese medicine, a pathogen can mean an unwelcome virus, bacteria, or fungus, but it can also mean an emotion. Here at the deepest level of the pulse we see the emergence of a pathological emotion, perhaps fear, which has caused the Constitutional Qi to become disrupted, creating a moving pulse, one that shifts from side to side. Emotions that are unresolved affect our organs, our gut, our digestion, creating a sense of imbalance and an inability to move forward with freedom. At the right side of the painting we see the emotions reaching a state of equilibrium and the resulting relaxing of the flow of Qi in the torso, creating a sense of comparative calm. Whatever is not resolved in this lifetime evaporates into the void of the spiritual universe, ready for resolution in a subsequent lifetime.

23. MOVING, VIBRATING

The Moving pulse is felt after the bone is palpated with 15 beans of pressure. It is a Hidden pulse that oscillates laterally and medially, indicating pathology of the Moving Qi of the Kidneys. It's sometimes called the Vibrating pulse, but I prefer not to use that term because it implies a buzzing quality and the frequency of vibration is not that at all—the pulse position oscillates with the beat of the pulse, one beat medial, one beat lateral, one beat medial, etc.

Feels like: The Moving pulse is quite distinctive. The beats oscillate steadily between two small areas within the area of contact. One area is closer to the radial artery and the other is closer to the radius.

Note: Sometimes I find this pulse without pressing into the bone, even up in the moderate or superficial levels. Invariably after closer examination I find that this means that the body is either requesting or would be receptive to an Eight Extraordinary channel treatment.

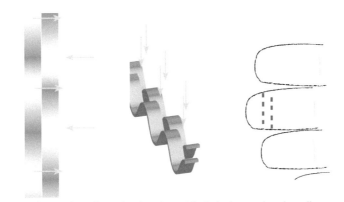

The moving pulse alternates back and forth between two locations on the finger.

24. NORMAL

The pulse has no remarkable features and feels healthy and full of Qi. A "Normal" pulse doesn't spill into the territory of another pulse, nor is it very isolated.

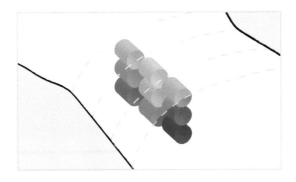

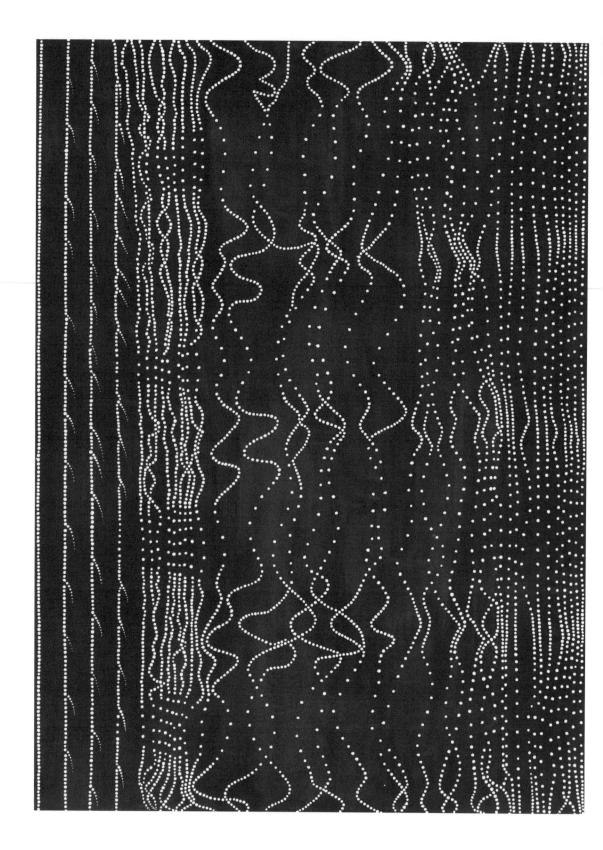

Earth Pulse

This painting shows the reception of Yang Qi (the warming and moving Qi of the Earth), its absorption into the sole of the foot at Bubbling Spring, and the resulting effervescence in the Blood and Qi. Yang Qi is consolidated at the deepest level of Qi since it is considered precious and to be treasured, and is meted out to the organs. It is this Qi that creates the Heart beat, the dance of the Blood, the movement of the mediumship of life. Yang Qi also forms the upper layer of Qi which transmits our feelings and intention, broadcasting our clear vision for the benefit of all.

25. SUPERFICIAL

This is the pulse most commonly mentioned in the *Mai Jing* because of the strong *Shang Han Lun* influence. The words superficial and floating are the same character in Chinese but in practice they are quite distinct. A Superficial pulse is a Tight pulse which is felt at between one and three beans of pressure. It indicates pathology, usually Wind-Cold, residing in the Wei level, that is, in the Sinew Channels while the body is unsupported by resources beneath that level. The Floating pulse is being pushed upward and therefore indicates an active immune response sufficiently supported by Fluids from the Ying Level.

Feels like: Approach the patient's pulse with the lightest of pressure (one bean of pressure). The Superficial pulse feels as though it is coming up almost out of the skin to meet your finger. When you press down on a Superficial pulse you see that the Tightness was only present at between one and three beans of pressure. There is no substance beneath the Superficial pulse pushing the pulse upward. This means Ying Qi and Yang are not supporting Wei Qi.

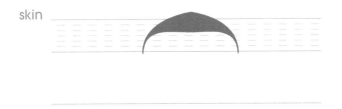

26. FLOATING

The Floating pulse is characterized by a discernible pressure that follows the finger up toward the surface from any level. It's characterized by an upward pressure against the finger as it is slowly lifted from one level to another. When you press down on a Floating pulse and then immediately relax the pressure on it, you receive confirmation that the pulse is being pushed up, that there is mediumship behind the pulse and that the body has the resources to move the pathology out. Injury recovery time is much shorter when the pulse is Floating rather than Superficial. The Floating pulse is discussed in Scroll 4 of the *Mai Jing*.
Floating Pulses in the Elderly: A Floating pulse that is also Long or Scattered indicates a chronic condition. These pulses are common in the elderly.

Feels like: As you lift a finger slowly from any level upward, each beat of the pulse is felt almost chasing the finger upward.

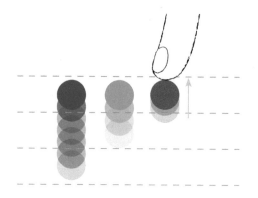

A pulse is floating when it follows your rising finger with pressure.
The terms applies to travel from any level upward to the Wei level.

26A. FLOODING, SURGING

A Flooding pulse is floating, full and rapid. It might also be big and long. The Flooding pulse indicates that Ying Qi is becoming deficient and unable to balance the warm, moving nature of Wei Qi. This causes the amount of heat at the surface to increase. In a Flooding pulse that is not very rapid, Blood may be coming to the surface to convert to Wei Qi, resulting in redness and heat, nosebleeds, bloodshot eyes and coughing of blood. Blood is becoming exuberant to finance Wei Qi as the body attempts to prevent something going deeper into the body. In *Shang Han Lun* terms this would be considered Heat in Yang Ming where Yang Qi is exuberant and there is Heat or Fire. The Flooding quality comes from the tension involved in squeezing the Ying up toward the Wei level. This extreme movement is not smooth and can result in a Rough pulse. A Flooding pulse can mean the Heart is moving Blood to expel Wind.

26B. HOLLOW, SCALLION

In a Scallion pulse, a matching tightness can be found in the deep and superficial levels, but there is no such sensation at the moderate level. The moderate level seems vacant as Ying Qi is not supporting Wei Qi. Fluids may need to be generated and the Spleen and Stomach may need to be supported. A Hollow pulse may indicate a loss of Blood. The Hollow pulse might also be Tight or Leathery on the superficial level, protecting against further depletion of resources.

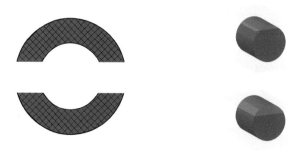

27. SOFT

The Soft pulse is a dynamic pulse. That is, it only shows itself when you are engaged, moving your finger. A Soft pulse can present in two ways. Either you find a Superficial pulse but as you push down on it a little it gives way, revealing that there is no substance under it, or you feel pressure upwards meaning that something is being expelled but the pulse doesn't have the integrity to push up all the way to the surface. There isn't enough mediumship to support Wei Qi. This pulse can be felt at the superficial or moderate levels, although a pulse that scatters at the deep level is also sometimes called Soft.

Comparison with Scattered: In general, the term Soft means that there is little integrity as you are pressing downward. The term Scattered means integrity is lacking as your finger is moving upward.

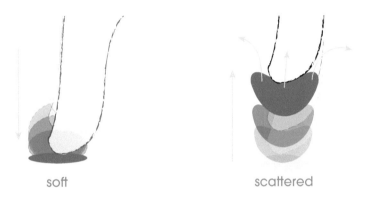

soft   scattered

28. URGENT

While examining an Urgent pulse your fingers simply don't want to stay in contact with the skin. Sometimes the Urgent pulse emits what feels like a tiny electric shock. This pulse may indicate an entitic invasion, or parasites. If the pulse shows urgency on a moderate level, this indicates that the problem is likely in one's own home. If the urgency is felt on the deep level, entitic invasion of the person is indicated.

Note: In my practice I find that the Urgent pulse is most often located in the Heart position. Needle GV-26 and moxa LU-11 and SP-1 to release an entity in the Sun Si Miao style.

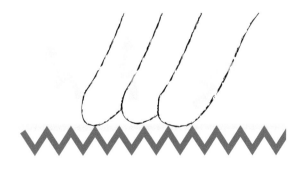

HASTY, KNOTTED AND INTERMITTENT

The following three irregular pulses show pathology at the Yuan level preventing Heart and Kidney communication. At the deep level, these pulses might hide and reappear. The regularity of the pulses is predicated on the strength and openness of the Heart's communication with the Kidneys; it is the microcosmic orbit that allows for things to be rhythmic. Hasty, Knotted and Intermittent pulses demonstrate that there is pathology obstructing the circuitous nature of this communication. Examining pulses in the Kidney position takes more time than those of any other pulse.

29. HASTY

The Hasty pulse indicates pathology at the Yuan level as Heat consumes the Jing. The pulse is Rapid and misses beats; it lacks steady rhythm.

30. KNOTTED

The Knotted pulse indicates pathology at the Yuan level. It is missing a beat at irregular intervals and is Slow. This pulse indicates that there is stagnation of Yin. This could be due to Cold, Yin or Yang deficiency, etc.

31. INTERMITTENT

The Intermittent pulse indicates pathology at the Yuan level. It misses a beat at regular or near-regular intervals but can be Slow or Rapid. It can appear normal unless you spend time in the chi position. The irregular pulse shows that something is being withheld, perhaps something is stagnant or even latent. Often this pulse emerges in patients who are confused about the direction of their life or who lack enthusiasm. The enthusiasm has leaked out and the flatness of the Heart causes gaps to appear in the chi position as the Kidneys try to rest and collect resources.

FREQUENTLY ASKED QUESTION

How is it possible for the pulse to beat at a different rate to the heart beat felt in the chest?
The pulses felt in the wrist (or elsewhere, distal to the heart) are not a simple result of the individual beats of the heart. At the various pulse locations all over the body (the carotid, the dorsalis pedis, the wrist) we are feeling the vibration of the radiation of Qi, of one's life force. The pulses we feel are a shimmering of Qi from all the viscera, not the sensation of the flow of blood in the arteries. The ancients discovered that close to the mouth of Qi (LU-9) existed a map of the vibrations emanating from the organs. The unique feelings we have in each of the six pulse positions are truly reflections of the Qi in those organs and in those media.

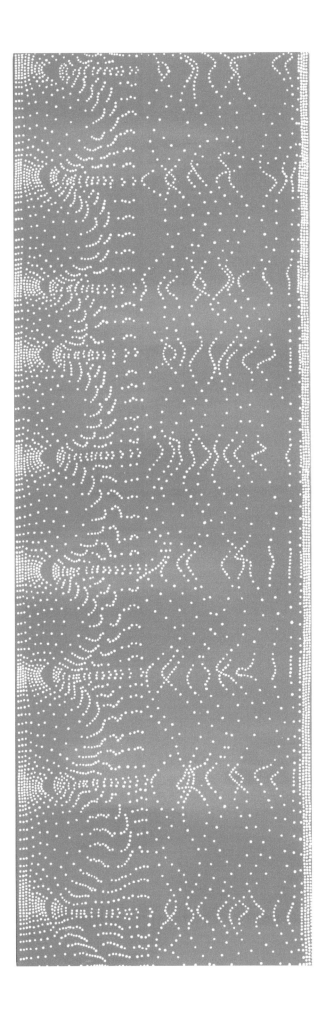

Hasty Pulse

The Hasty Pulse feels irregular and rapid. Heat feels as though it's radiating from the Yuan level. The Heart skips a beat as the Heart and the Kidneys are not in alignment. The Kidneys provide the Will to go forward, to pursue one's true path which is revealed in the desires of the Heart. If the Mind has a differing opinion, a blockage is created in the Middle Jiao, forming an obstacle to Heart-Kidney communication. The Hasty Pulse has a frantic quality. The practitioner offers calm and transmits inspiration to relax into self-discovery and self-acceptance.

Intermittent Pulse

This painting shows the irregularity detected in the pulse when the Heart and Kidneys are not communicating effectively. The Kidneys store the plans for the playing out of life's purpose. The Heart communicates down to the Kidneys, obtains data relating to our personal life's purpose and relates it back up into the chest where the Lungs contribute inspiration received from Heaven. The Heart resonates in a new way with these communications and is able to shine its light outward, with joy and quiet excitement as life is being lived meaningfully. When the mind interrupts this communication with it's habitual limiting thought about what is and what isn't possible, the pulse becomes interrupted. The practitioner sees a gentle invitation to remind the patient to remember why they are here, and to act on it for their benefit and the benefit of all. When the mind relinquishes its protest, the pulse resumes its regularity.

PREFACE TO CHAPTERS 3 AND 4

To understand Dynamic Pulses, it is important to have a clear feeling of the remarkably vast, spacious quality of the pulse. When we first start learning pulses many of us are puzzled that anyone could feel so much detail because the pulses seem such a tiny, shallow part of the anatomy. But the distance we can explore in the pulse is enormously spacious when examined from the surface of the skin down to the level of the bone.

When I teach pulse diagnosis in the classroom, the aspect I need to correct most often is the depth of the fingers at the pulse. When beginning to learn pulse depths, most people think they are deep in the pulse when they are only at about nine beans of pressure. Twelve beans is a long way into the pulse. Fifteen beans requires a considerable pressure.

The following exercise illustrates the surprisingly substantial depth of the pulse. Please take yourself through it before proceeding.

EXERCISE TO EXPERIENCE THE ENTIRE DEPTH EXAMINED IN THE TAKING OF THE PULSE

1. Assume the position of taking the pulses on either your own or a patient's wrist, but don't yet make contact with the skin.

2. Very slowly, allow the tiniest amount of the skin of your three fingers to make contact with the tiniest amount, the very surface of the patient's (or your own) skin. You will almost not be touching the skin. Pretend you are barely touching the most delicate butterfly wing. This depth is defined as one bean of pressure.

3. As slowly as possible, add the smallest amount of pressure, almost none at all. Now a bit more, and a bit more. Over a period of about a minute, extremely slowly, move your fingers down into the pulse as slowly as you possibly can.

4. At some point, perhaps about half way through the minute, you'll be aware that you have made contact with the radial artery. Keep going very slowly until you feel you are in the middle of the artery. This depth is defined as nine beans of pressure.

5. Quite a while after that, you'll feel that if you keep going, you'll stop the flow of blood in the radial artery. Keep going.

6. The flow of blood will stop and very soon after that you'll become aware of the hardness of the bone. Slowly go into the bone. Then keep going until you feel you are compressing the bone a little. This depth is defined as fifteen beans of pressure.

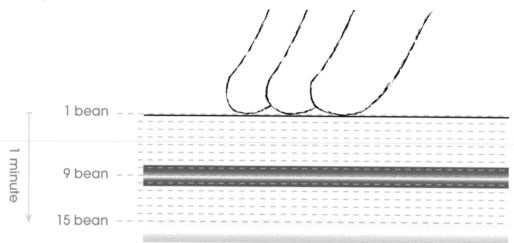

If this exercise is done slowly it's difficult not to be utterly staggered by the magnitude of the distance your finger can travel in the action of moving from the superficial skin through to pressing into the bone. What seems like a small distance becomes a vast arena offering a whole world of information. It's remarkable. In traversing that distance, with practice, it is possible to answer a plethora of diagnostic questions.

CHAPTER 3

PROBING DYNAMIC PULSES AND ORGAN FUNCTION

From the pulses we are able to discern how well an organ is functioning. As soon as you touch the patient's pulses an interchange begins. Often a pulse feels as though it would like to behave in a different way. By applying focused mental intention the pulses can begin to realign themselves. This doesn't mean we are imposing judgment; rather, it means that the change the pulse is trying to make is being honored and facilitated by the practitioner's intention. Treatment begins before any needles are inserted. If you cannot get a pulse to change by concentrating on it and willing it to change, the condition is in the organ itself, not its associated channel. This section describes the functions of the organs and their detection through probing dynamic pulses. This technique involves varying the depth of an individual finger at an individual position (cun, guan or chi) and noting the response in the pulse at that same position. Whether one chooses probing pulses or directional pulses or both to detect organ function is a matter of personal preference. Some organ functions, however, are best felt using directional pulses. These include the communication between Heart to Kidneys, Kidneys to Heart, Kidneys to Lungs and Lungs to Kidneys.

Vocabulary qualifying the sensations in the pulses is explained in Chapter 2.

The Triple Pressure Imperative

All discussion about diagnosis in this manual involves pressure on all three pulse positions. Pulses are not read with pressure applied only to one position because the organ systems are never functioning alone. We always are mindful of the relationships. The default finger depth for the cun and guan positions is the moderate level. The default finger position for the chi position is the deep level. When reading the Liver pulse, for example, the focus is on the guan position while the finger at the cun position is at the moderate level and the finger at the chi position is at the deep level. If the fingers were lifted off the two positions not being considered, the function of the organ being examined would not be clearly shown. The pressure provided by the "idle" fingers simulates the natural internal pressure of the entire physiological system, enabling the pulse taker to get a true picture of the organ in its working context.

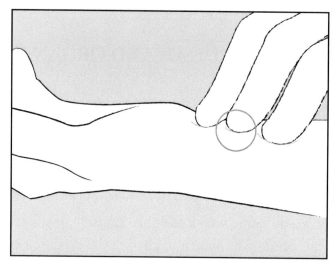

Pressure is maintained in all three positions at all times, even if
the practitioner is only focussing on one finger. This simulates the interconnected
internal pressures of a working system.

LUNG FUNCTION AND ITS PRESENCE IN THE PULSES

The Lung pulse should be strong at the moderate level and should float and disperse, following your finger up to the surface. At the chi position, the Kidneys engender Yang Qi which manifests in the cun position, the Lung pulse. If you push down on the Lung pulse, you should feel it pushing up even more at six beans; it should feel more vibrant. This is part of the floating quality. If it doesn't have a floating quality, then the Spleen needs to be treated to support Wei Qi, because Spleen Yang supports Lung function, or, in another way of seeing, Spleen Yang conducts Kidney Yang Qi up to the Lungs, along with the products of digestion, to be distributed by the Lungs in their role of dispersing. This is what we are looking for in reading the vibrancy of the Lung pulse at six beans, to see whether it has healthy qualities of floating and dispersing.

The Lungs function in order to:
1. Govern Qi
2. Descend Qi
3. Effuse/Diffuse/Disperse Qi
4. Rectify Qi
5. Moisten
6. Move Blood
7. Govern the capacity to let go and forgive or let go and accept.

1. GOVERN QI.

The Lung channel begins at CV-12. A morsel of Yuan Qi stirs the Lungs to fully expand to receive Qi. The Lungs govern Qi in the sense that they receive Qi and let go of Qi.

Pulse Sensation: The moderate level of the pulse should feel strong. This means the connection to the origin of Qi is strong. The Lung pulse should float to confirm that the Lungs can let go of Qi during respiration.

2. DESCEND QI.

The Lungs descend Qi to the Kidneys. This descension of Qi enables the opening of the Lower Jiao for conception, menstruation, urination and defecation. The Qi of the Lungs descends to the Kidneys to fan Ming Men, Life Gate at GV-4. This means that the Qi of Heaven permeates us, awakening our destiny within us.

Pulse Sensation: As you press down from the moderate level into the deep level, the Lung pulse should become stronger and fuller at the deep level.

3. EFFUSE/DIFFUSE/DISPERSE QI.

The primary focus of Lung Qi is exhalation. The Lungs are the key organ for letting go of Qi.

Pulse Sensation: The Lung pulse should float. There should be a sense of energy rising. As you release pressure from the pulse at the moderate level, there should be a steady, consistent pressure behind your finger pushing it up to the top of the Wei level. It should float. It is normal for the Lung pulse to be scattered as your finger moves through the Wei level; this is a mark of diffusion.

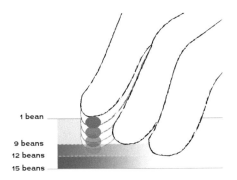

4. RECTIFY QI.

This means that a patient is able to discern what is right for him or her, and what is not.

Pulse Sensation: The pulse is strong in the moderate level. It should not be wiry, thin, beady or slippery. This means that the origin of the Lung Channel, CV-12, is strong. There is clarity in the gut generating a knowing of what is right and wrong for the individual. This clarity is unobstructed by dampness.

5. MOISTEN.

The Lungs move Fluids and Blood to moisten.

Pulse Sensation: The pulse is wide at the superficial level indicating that the Lungs are able to move mediumship. The pulse should not be rapid. If the Lungs do not have good width they are not receiving sufficient Fluids from the Middle Jiao. The Spleen ascends these Fluids from the Stomach. The Lungs then descend Yin to the Kidneys. The Lungs descend to the Lower Jiao to moisten the Large Intestine.

6. MOVE BLOOD.

The dispersing function of the Lungs indicates how well they are moving Blood.

Pulse Sensation: This is evident in the degree to which the Lung pulse floats from the moderate to the superficial level.

7. GOVERN THE CAPACITY TO LET GO AND FORGIVE OR LET GO AND ACCEPT.

The Lungs release not only External Pathogenic Factors (EPFs) but control feelings of vulnerability, insecurity, injustice, and the sense of morality.

Pulse Sensation: The pulse should not be wiry or beady. A wiry pulse shows that something cannot be let go. A beady pulse tells us that long-term Phlegm has obstructed the Lungs and their capacity to let go. The Lung pulse should float without feeling slippery. As you release pressure from the pulse at the moderate level, there should be a steady, consistent pressure behind your finger pushing it up to the top of the Wei level. It might scatter as it reaches the Wei level.

PATHOLOGICAL QUALITIES OF THE LUNG PULSE

Generally, the Lungs show pathology if the pulse is not strong at the moderate level, does not disperse, and is beady, tight, wiry or slippery.

HEART FUNCTION AND ITS PRESENCE IN THE PULSES

The Heart pulse should feel full as you raise your finger and relaxed as you push down on it. This means that there is enough Blood for the conduction of experiences and excitement and for the creation of reality. The Heart should have no Yin factors. Yin factors (Damp and Phlegm) hamper its freedom. The Heart should only have Yang pulses. The Heart nourishes the Shen because it is naturally curious and excited. The Heart pulse should be excited, bold and strong, but not rapid.

The Heart functions to:

      1. Govern circulation and move Blood to the periphery

      2. Invigorate Blood.

      3. Open to the tongue.

      4. Share love and joy.

      5. House the Shen.

      6. Open to the eyes.

1. GOVERN CIRCULATION AND MOVE BLOOD TO THE PERIPHERY

The optimal circulation of blood allows us to engage in the world and to experience the excitement, joy and interaction the world offers us and that the Heart seeks. The Blood of the Heart seeks human interaction.

Pulse Sensation: The pulse should be strong and full on the moderate level. As the finger is lifted from the deep level, through the moderate level and into the superficial level, the pulse should become stronger and stronger because blood is coming out to the world. The Heart pulse should become full as the finger is on the way up and relaxed as the finger is on the way down.

2. INVIGORATE BLOOD.

Pulse Sensation: The pulse should be strongest at the moderate level, the level of Blood.

3. OPEN TO THE TONGUE.

The Heart opens to the Tongue in order to share joy and express excitement.

Pulse Sensation: The pulse should scatter slightly as it floats to the superficial level from the moderate level.

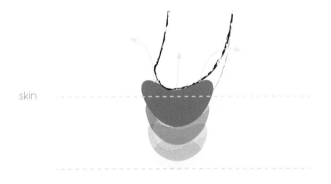

skin

4. SHARE LOVE AND JOY.

This includes the joy experienced in satisfying curiosity and the joy experienced in sharing joy itself. I have found this scattering quality very reliable in determining the patient's level of optimism.

Pulse Sensation: On the superficial level, the Heart pulse scatters slightly, demonstrating the patient's willingness to spread love and joy.

5. HOUSE THE SHEN.

The deep level of the Heart pulse is the location of the retreat of the Shen. Sometimes this pulse will vibrate indicating this retreat is pathological. But a Shen's retreating nature might also be intrinsic. The deep level illustrates the degree to which the Kidney receives the Yang Qi from the Heart and is able to calm the Shen; the Yang anchors the Shen.

Pulse Sensation: An anchored Shen will show in the deep level of the Heart pulse as relaxed and replete, or even gentle and soft. In this case, the soft pulse is not pathological. An anchored Shen can also show as a Heart pulse that is very slightly tight only at the superficial level. This very superficial tightness is holding the Shen in place. If the pulse at the deep level of the Heart is not relaxed, the patient is unable to calm his or her own Shen, or can't sleep.

6. OPEN TO THE EYES.

To convey excitement and enthusiasm.

Pulse Sensation: The Heart pulse floats. (It follows your finger as you lift it.)

Note that you might find that the Heart pulse has moved up to the superficial level because the patient is delighted to find that you are interested in them. A heart-to-heart conversation, which can be a part of an acupuncture treatment encounter moves the Heart.

PATHOLOGICAL QUALITIES OF THE HEART PULSE

A *wiry Heart pulse* indicates the Heart is constrained. This can be caused by Dampness or Phlegm. Or the patient is knowingly or unknowingly agreeing to a limitation being placed on the amount of joy their Heart is allowed to express.

A *tight pulse* shows obstruction or stagnation in the Heart for similar reasons but at an earlier stage. Sometimes, however, the Heart pulse can be a little tight on the superficial level as the Shen is held in place. This is not pathological.

A *rapid Heart pulse* is showing that there is too much excitement causing Heat. The Heat is in turn preventing the natural nourishment and fulfillment that comes from that very excitement. If the Heart is rapid as it scatters, there is too much stimulation, enough to negatively impact intelligence.

An urgent Heart pulse can indicate the presence of an entity.

A slippery Heart pulse, especially at the moderate level, means the Spleen is not able to ascend enough Yang to enable the Stomach to adequately ripen and rot; Phlegm in the gut then moves up with the red substance as the red substance is ascended from the Spleen to the Heart. The Phlegm should have been expectorated by the Lungs but the Lungs might have been weak or are currently weak.

SPLEEN FUNCTION AND ITS PRESENCE IN THE PULSES

The Spleen pulse naturally is strong with integrity at its borders. It is slightly slippery at the moderate level but not slippery at all in the deep level.

The Spleen functions to:
1. Transform and Transport.
2. Ascend Kidney Yang to the Stomach.
3. Ascend the Pure Yang of the Stomach to the sensory orifices.
4. Ascend Blood to the Heart.
5. Manage blood.
6. Control the Mind.
7. Produce Gu Qi (along with the Stomach).
8. Resolve Dampness and Discharge Dampness.
9. Control the four limbs.
10. Rectify Qi in the Lungs.
11. Support Kidneys in Consolidating Qi.
12. Harmonize with the Stomach.

1. TRANSFORM AND TRANSPORT.

The Spleen maintains fluid metabolism via the process of transformation during the initial process of separation which occurs in the Stomach. The Spleen allows for the extraction of Qi from the fine particles of digestion.

Pulse Sensation: The pulse is strong at the moderate level. The Spleen pulse is naturally very slightly slippery at the moderate level which is the level of the Stomach organ. This is because the Stomach must ripen and rot in order for the Spleen to be able to transform the food. In other words, to be able to cook food (for the Spleen to be able to transform food) one must have the right amount of water (fluids provided by the Stomach). A slippery pulse at the deep level in the Spleen position is pathological, however, because it indicates Dampness in the Spleen itself.

2. ASCEND KIDNEY YANG TO THE STOMACH.

The Spleen provides the ascending movement that brings the Yang of the Kidneys into the digestive tract. This is the Yang required to transform and transport nourishment. Concurrently, the Stomach descends the Qi through the digestive tract.

Pulse Sensation: The descending function of the Stomach is felt as your finger moves from the superficial level to the moderate level; it should become stronger. The ascending function of the Spleen is felt as you move down further to the next level, that is, as you press down from the moderate to the deep level the Spleen pulse should become slightly stronger as you press down.

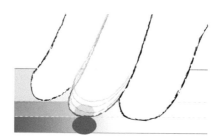

3. ASCEND THE PURE YANG OF THE STOMACH TO THE SENSORY ORIFICES.

The Spleen ascends the pure thin fluids of the Stomach to the sensory orifices so that there is a mediumship to register sight, sound and taste, then to imprint those sensations on the sensory orifices. Without that fluid, life is perceived to be dull.

Pulse Sensation: The ascending function of the Spleen is felt as a slight increase in strength as you move down from the moderate to the deep level.

4. ASCEND BLOOD TO THE HEART.

The Spleen brings the red substance up to the Heart for the finalization of the production of Blood. The Spleen has to store enough red substance at the Stomach in order to transfer it to the Heart for finalization so it can be sent to the Liver to be stored. This blood is delivered to the Liver by the Liver's Jue Yin partner, the Pericardium.

Pulse Sensation: This is a subset of the ascending function of the Spleen. The Spleen pulse should feel slightly stronger as you press from the moderate level to the deep level.

5. MANAGE BLOOD.

The action of holding Blood in its banks is conducted by the Spleen. The Spleen prevents the leakage of Blood.

Pulse Sensation: There is a certain sense of healthy containment in the Spleen pulse. The walls of the vessel in the moderate level feel shored up without being tight. There is good definition in the borders of the Spleen pulse.

6. CONTROL THE MIND.

One of the Spleen's roles is to think about things that are meaningful to the Heart. This is what it really means to bank the Blood. Concentration on these thoughts is in parallel with the literal management or concentration of Blood in the vessels. If thoughts are in keeping with the openness of the Heart, the Spleen has integrity and there will be no hemorrhages or varicosities. The Spleen tempers excessive thinking and resolves that which afflicts the Heart. The Spleen elevates the light that the Heart emanates.

Pulse Sensation: The Spleen pulse has integrity at its sides, feels stable and contained; the walls of the artery feel firm. There is a sense of buoyancy in the moderate level.

7. PRODUCE GU QI (ALONG WITH THE STOMACH).

Gu Qi is a term which means the combination of digestive Qi contained in the chyme and the red substance; in other words, the production of Qi and Blood.

Pulse Sensation: This is felt in the width of the moderate level of the Spleen pulse.

8. RESOLVE DAMPNESS AND DISCHARGE DAMPNESS.

The Spleen resolves Dampness by ensuring there is sufficient Yang being sent upward from the Kidneys to ensure complete digestion.

Pulse Sensation: This function is felt as a slight increase in the strength of the Spleen pulse as the finger presses from the moderate to the deep levels. The Spleen pulse is devoid of slipperiness at the deep level if the Spleen's performance of this function is meeting the demands of the body.

9. CONTROL THE FOUR LIMBS.

The Spleen is responsible for the distribution of Qi to the four limbs, keeping them animated and keeping the hands and feet warm. The four limbs also represent acting out of compassion, walking and moving the arms in order to act out one's life purpose, certain in one's values and beliefs.

Pulse Sensation: Again, the up and out motion of Spleen Qi is felt as a strengthening of the pulse between the moderate and deep levels.

10. RECTIFY QI IN THE LUNGS.

The Spleen rectifies Lung Qi by elevating thoughts to the Lungs to enable the Lungs to let go of pathology (in this case, Phlegm). The Spleen elevates thought to the Lungs to spur them to let go of the phlegm, to forgive, to accept, to let go of afflicting memories.

Pulse Sensation: This is felt as a combination of the ascending vector of the Spleen pulse to the Lungs and the immediate dispersal of Lung Qi, seen as a floating pulse in the Lung position.

11. SUPPORT KIDNEYS IN CONSOLIDATING QI.

The Spleen supports the Kidneys through focus on thoughts that promote self-esteem. The Spleen's elemental partner, the Stomach, then descends this Qi to the Kidneys.

Pulse Sensation: In the right guan position, as you press down from the superficial level to the moderate level, the pulse should become stronger. This shows that the Stomach is descending. At the same time, the Spleen pulse feels as though it has integrity; it ascends confidently. This is demonstrated as the Spleen pulse offers resistance as it is pressed from the moderate to the deep level.

12. HARMONIZE WITH THE STOMACH.

The Spleen ascends Qi, and in so doing enables its elemental partner the Stomach to descend Qi.

Pulse Sensation: Descension of the Stomach is demonstrated as your finger goes from superficial to moderate and experiences a strengthening of the pulse. The ascension of the Spleen is shown as a resistance against the finger that emerges as the finger moves from the moderate level to deep level. If these two sensations match, the Spleen and the Stomach are harmonized.

PATHOLOGICAL QUALITIES OF THE SPLEEN PULSE

Generally, the Lungs show pathology if the pulse is not strong at the moderate level, and is tight, wiry, or very slippery

LIVER FUNCTION AND ITS PRESENCE IN THE PULSES

The Liver pulse is naturally slightly tight at the moderate level, especially between six and nine beans. Sometimes it is tighter in women because its principal function is to gather and store Blood. It should not be wiry, as that would indicate stagnation. There is a natural softness at the deep level. The pulse does not become thinner as it is pressed more deeply, especially when pressed beyond 12 beans. The Liver pulse maintains integrity throughout the entire depth of the pulse until you reach beyond 12 beans when it starts to disintegrate as its blood is broken down to nourish Jing-Essence. It shows ascension in moving up with your finger when you raise it and descension by pressing up against your finger as you move your finger downward. The Liver pulse should not scatter, as that indicates Wind in the Liver.

The Liver functions to:

1. Regulate Qi.
2. Engender Heart Qi.
3. Engender Heart Blood.
4. Course or Spread the Qi.
5. Regulate the smooth flow of Qi.
6. Store Blood.
7. Discharge Dampness, especially Damp-Heat.
8. Bring Blood to the Sinews.
9. Bring Blood to the Brain.
10. Open to the Eyes.
11. Plan.
12. The Liver stores the Hun (the collective unconscious) and store memories
13. Nourish the Kidneys.
14. Nourish the structure, hair and nails.
15. Send Blood to the Kidneys to foster self-worth.
16. Bring Blood to the Lower Jiao for Fertility and Creativity.

1. REGULATE QI.

Pulse Sensation: The vectors of ascension and descension are felt equally; as you lift your finger, the pulse follows the finger up and as you apply more pressure the pulse continues to have integrity, although it will soften in the deep level. This is normal.

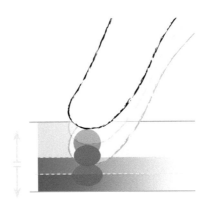

2. ENGENDER HEART QI.

Liver Blood not only becomes Jing-Essence or Kidney Yin, it also becomes Heart Qi. The Liver gives the Heart the resources it needs to find things interesting, to find life interesting. The Heart and the Liver both go to the eyes. The eyes reveal new things to the Heart and the Liver provides the resources to create achievements in relation to what is seen. Heart Qi draws upon Liver Blood, using the Liver's resources to create action and bring about the realization of one's destiny or life's purpose.

Pulse Sensation: As you lift your finger slowly from the moderate level, the pulse energetically follows you.

3. ENGENDER HEART BLOOD.

Pulse Sensation: As you lift your finger within the moderate level, the pulse feels wide and plentiful.

4. COURSE OR SPREAD THE QI.

The Liver is responsible for the spreading of Qi through both Yin and Yang Sinews, which in turn control all the smooth muscle and the exterior.

Pulse Sensation: The Liver is slightly tight, but not wiry, and is able to follow your finger up and remain strong as you push your finger back down into the pulse.

5. REGULATE THE SMOOTH FLOW OF QI.

The Liver controls the diaphragm, which must be relaxed in order to maintain the smooth flow of Qi. A stagnated Liver can oppress the diaphragm.

Pulse Sensation: The Liver pulse might feel slightly tight but the top of the pulse comes up into your finger. It is not circumferentially tight.

6. STORE BLOOD.

The Liver stores blood. Most of one's Blood is returned to the Liver with every heart beat during sleep.

Pulse Sensation: The Liver is shown to be storing Blood when the Liver pulse is slightly tight, or tight between six and nine beans of pressure. To store Blood there must be Qi at the Liver position; it cannot be weak.

7. DISCHARGE DAMPNESS, ESPECIALLY DAMP-HEAT.

The Liver usually discharges Dampness by generating diarrhea. This is its detoxifying method. The Gallbladder is used to hasten this discharge and move the stagnation.

Pulse Sensation: The Liver shows it is able to discharge Dampness when the pulse is felt to maintain its integrity in the moderate level and soften when pressed to the deep level. This is normal.

8. BRING BLOOD TO THE SINEWS.

Pulse Sensation: The pulse follows your finger upward from the moderate level to within the upper level of the pulse.

9. BRING BLOOD TO THE BRAIN.

Liver Blood nourishes the brain via the internal branch that connects the Liver to the brain and terminates at GV-20.

Pulse Sensation: The pulse follows your finger as you move from the moderate level up to three beans of pressure. The Liver is ascending Blood to the brain.

10. OPEN TO THE EYES.

The Liver opens to the eyes via the first branch of the Liver Primary Channel.

Pulse Sensation: The pulse follows your finger as you move from the moderate level up to three beans of pressure.

11. PLAN.

The Liver stores Blood which in turn stores memory. This enables the Liver to plan. (The Liver plans, planning is Yin; the Gallbladder is the decision maker, deciding is Yang.)

Pulse Sensation: The Liver pulse is slightly tight. It is not wiry; a stagnated Liver cannot be flexible enough to plan.

12. HOUSE THE HUN.

The Liver stores the Hun (the collective unconscious) and store memories or images of the past, present and future.

Pulse Sensation: The pulse is slightly tight between nine and six beans of pressure. The sides of the pulse have integrity.

13. NOURISH THE KIDNEYS.

Blood from the Liver nourishes the Kidneys. This is one of the few ways postnatal Qi nourishes Jing-Essence.

Pulse Sensation: There must be Qi available in order to store Blood. A weak Liver pulse indicates that there is insufficient Qi to store Blood and so Liver Blood cannot be nourishing the Kidneys. If the Liver pulse is weak on the deep level, the Liver is not supporting the Essence and the structure. At 12 beans there should be softness in the pulse. Beyond that the pulse should almost feel as though it is disintegrating as Blood breaks apart to nourish the Essence. The Liver softens the Blood so that it can become Jing.

Note: (The softness described above should not be confused with weakness. The soft pulse that is weak is the one that is felt just beneath a floating pulse, indicating that Wei Qi is not being supported by Fluids.)

14. NOURISH THE STRUCTURE, HAIR AND NAILS.

Pulse Sensation: At 12 beans of pressure the pulse is not at all weak. If at this deep level it is weak, frail, empty or minute, the Liver is not supporting the structure, the hair or the nails. The weakness indicates the Liver has inadequate Qi which is required to store Blood and to move that Blood down to the Kidneys to support Jing-Essence.

15. SEND BLOOD TO THE KIDNEYS TO FOSTER SELF-WORTH.

Self-esteem is a function of Jing-Essence as it is stored in the Kidneys. Jing is replenished through postnatal Qi as Liver Blood nourishes Jing.

Pulse Sensation: At 12 beans there should be softness in the pulse and just beyond that the pulse should almost feel as though it is disintegrating as Blood breaks apart to nourish Jing-Essence. The Liver softens the Blood so that it can become Jing.

16. BRING BLOOD TO THE LOWER JIAO FOR FERTILITY AND CREATIVITY.

A shortage of Liver Blood moving to the genitalia to create Kidney Yin results in impotence, infertility and a lack of creativity.

Pulse Sensation: At 12 beans there should be a soft quality. (Soft does not mean weak.) At 12 beans you should begin to feel a meshing of the Blood and Jing levels. This is the juncture at which the Blood becomes Jing-Essence. If there's a melding here and a concurrent softening, the Blood is becoming denser, becoming Yin. The pulse should break apart when pressing deeper than 12 beans.

PATHOLOGICAL QUALITIES OF THE LIVER PULSE

A wiry pulse indicates stagnation of Liver Qi. The Liver is not storing Blood. Stagnation of the Liver also prevents the smooth flow of Qi and many other Liver functions. A wiry pulse can result from long term tightness from Cold. The impact of Cold on the Liver pulse can be very strong but it is not to be mistaken for strength; it is merely extreme tightness and the fight that has ensued to break up that Cold and push it out to the exterior. Extreme tightness can indicate late Shao Yin or Jue Yin pathology. Initially the pulse could be slow also, but in the long term it can be wiry. Wiry pulses show that Liver Blood cannot nourish the Heart or the Kidneys. Ultimately this can lead to a lack of interest in learning and in life as the Heart is not nourished. This can affect the patient's sense of self-worth and lead to shyness, timidity and apprehension, doubt and uncertainty. Moxa LR-12 to break up Cold in the Liver. Note that wiry should not be confused with tight. A wiry pulse is circumferentially tight; a tight pulse is tight at the sides.

A *thin Liver pulse* indicates the Liver is not storing enough Blood to be able to nourish the Heart and Kidneys.

A *rapid Liver pulse.* The Liver pulse should not be rapid. Heat would then be free to rise to the Heart.

A *slow Liver pulse.* The Liver pulse should not be slow. This would show that the Liver is stagnated and unable to effectively move Blood up or down.

A *scattered Liver pulse* indicates that internal Wind is present. Wind needs to be coursed or subdued. (If the Hun is not stable, calm the Shen with GB-9 and GB-13, even technique.)

A *floating Liver pulse* indicates that Yang is floating. Yang needs to be subdued or anchored.

A *Liver pulse* that is full in the superficial level indicates Yang is not anchored.

A *weak Liver pulse* shows that the Liver is not able to store Blood.

A *slippery Liver pulse* indicates an imbalance between the Liver and the Spleen. Treat the Spleen since the Spleen is not controlling Damp.

A *choppy Liver pulse* indicates the Liver is attempting to astringe (tighten its Qi around) Blood but there is insufficient Blood to store. This feels like an accordion under your finger as it dilates and tightens, dilates and tightens.

KIDNEY FUNCTION AND ITS PRESENCE IN THE PULSES

The Kidney pulses are felt at the deep level where they naturally are slightly tight, as their principal function is to conserve Jing-Essence. They should feel strong and full.

When pressure is released from the deep level, the pulse should follow your finger to the cusp of the moderate level. The Kidney pulse should feel strong there as well.

A Kidney pulse felt at the superficial level is pathological. To a lesser degree a Kidney pulse felt at the moderate level is also pathological.

The Kidney Yin pulse, felt on the left side, is called the stone pulse; it is naturally tight, slow and heavy as it seeks to conserve Jing-Essence. The slowness is not to be confused with Cold. Cold is simply the nature of Jing, and is supposed to be conserved and used sparingly.

The Kidney Yang pulse which is on the right should be faster than its Yin partner. Kidney Yang is the foundation of warmth, movement and enthusiasm for life. It provides the movement needed to disseminate Jing-Essence to the Bladder Shu points, maintaining the minute-to-minute functioning of the organs. A rapid Kidney Yang pulse at the deep level might not be pathological but might indicate great enthusiasm for life. The Kidney Yang pulse should simply be strong. The Kidney Yang pulse should not be any more than slightly tight, if it is tight at all. If it is tight it may be acting to prevent leakage.

The Kidney pulse can be slightly soft when the patient is in deep contemplation or in a state of deep relaxation.

The Kidneys Function to:
1. Control Reproduction.
2. Control Growth, Decay and Decline.
3. House the Zhi-Will.
4. Consolidate and Secure the Essence.
5. Maintain the bones, structure, shape and form.
6. Regulate the Waterways.
7. Receive Qi.
8. Control the lower orifices.
9. Disseminate Yang Qi.

1. CONTROL REPRODUCTION.
The Kidneys secure the Essence, ensuring the storage of the resources necessary for procreation.
Pulse Sensation: The Kidney Yin pulse (left) is slightly tight.

2. CONTROL GROWTH, DECAY AND DECLINE.
The Kidneys secure the Jing-Essence so that Jing is not wasted, its decline not hastened. This optimizes the availability of Jing for the carrying out of growth bound in one's destiny.
Pulse Sensation: The Kidney Yin pulse (left) is slightly tight.

3. HOUSE THE ZHI-WILL.

The Zhi-Will is what encourages us to be who we truly are, rather than what society might dictate. The role of the Zhi is to navigate the true path of destiny and to ensure that we are true to ourselves.

Pulse Sensation: As you press more into the deep level the Kidney pulses should become stronger.

4. CONSOLIDATE AND SECURE THE ESSENCE.

The security of the Jing-Essence is dependent on one's endorsement of oneself. The Jing is secure if one can squarely say to oneself that they appreciate themselves, that they have a real love of the self. It is impossible to be true to oneself, to be authentic, if there is not love of the self. If there is self-loathing, or if there is the underlying feeling of shame about who one is, the Jing is consumed. Fire runs rampant as it is unbalanced and burning the Jing.

Pulse Sensation: As you press deeper into the deep level the Kidney pulse should become stronger. It should not become stronger as you raise your finger to the moderate level. That would indicate there is insufficient Qi to hold or to move the Yin down. This applies to the Yang and the Yin Kidney pulses.

5. MAINTAIN THE BONES, STRUCTURE, SHAPE AND FORM.

The Kidneys govern the way Jing-Essence is meted out to become our structure.

Pulse Sensation: As you press deeper into the deep level the Kidney pulse should become stronger.

6. REGULATE THE WATERWAYS.

The Kidneys determine how rapidly water will flow and change from a liquid state to a more solid state as it become Jing-Essence. (This movement is also regulated by the Yang Qi of Triple Heater and the Bladder Channel.) Triple Heater regulates the temperature of water, lowering it to allow water to become Jing and raising it to enable it to become Qi. During this process, turbid water must be moved so that it does not decay; Kidney Yang provides the movement for this process.

Pulse Sensation: The right Kidney pulse is strong and energetic in the deep level. It has good width.

7. RECEIVE QI.

The Kidneys are responsible for the reception of Qi. In the Kidney position, the reception of Stomach Qi and Lung Qi is felt.

Pulse Sensation: You might feel something in the moderate level of the Kidney pulse as you are diagnosing the reception of Qi. This is because the moderate level is the level of postnatal Qi and your focus is on the movement of Qi from that level down to the Kidneys. But during the process of moving your finger down from the moderate level to the deep level of the Kidney pulse, that is, from nine beans down to 15 beans of pressure, the pulse should become strong and fuller. This shows that the contract of life is accepted and the Qi of Heaven and of Humanity is accepted. Note that the emergence of the fullness and strength is not evident at 15 beans of pressure, but evident during the journey your finger makes from nine beans to 15 beans.

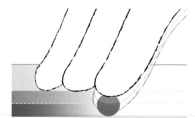

If the Lungs and Stomach are not descending, it means the Lungs and Stomach are not nourishing Kidney Qi. The Lungs and the Stomach are the postnatal receptors and they must both descend to support Kidney Qi. It is important to determine which of the two organs is not descending and then to treat that organ's function.

8. CONTROL THE LOWER ORIFICES.
The Kidneys control the urethra and anus.
Pulse Sensation: The Kidney Yang pulse (right) feels solid and anchored in the deep position. Its borders are well-defined.

9. DISSEMINATE YANG QI.
Kidney Yang is the foundation of the temperament. Ming Men supports the carrying out of a life's mandate. The Kidneys provide the Yang Qi to the Triple Heater to enable the dissemination of Jing-Essence to the Bladder Shu points which in turn transport that Jing to the organs for the expression of life.
Pulse Sensation: The pulse is anchored in the deep level and is not floating and scattered. As you release pressure from the deep to the bottom of the moderate level the pulse follows you but remains strong.

PATHOLOGICAL QUALITIES OF THE KIDNEY PULSE
A weak Kidney pulse shows the Kidney is unable to consolidate Jing-Essence.

A *rapid left Kidney (Yin) pulse* shows that Jing-Essence is being rapidly combusted.
A *wiry Kidney pulse* shows there is stagnation of the Jing-Essence; Jing is not being disseminated.

A *scattered Kidney Yang pulse* indicates escaping Yang.

A *floating Kidney pulse* in either position also means Yang is escaping.

A *slow, wiry pulse* in the Kidney Yang pulse can indicate Cold or stagnation.

A *slow Kidney Yang pulse* shows Cold or stagnation of Yang Qi. The Kidney Yang pulse should not have a quality that hampers movement.

A *tight Kidney Yang pulse* indicates that a Yin factor is hampering the movement of Yang.

A *floating, tight Kidney pulse* means the body is trying to stem leakage of Jing-Essence or Yin. As it escapes, Zong-Ancestral-Gathering Qi tries to anchor the Qi back down, making the pulse floating and tight.

YANG-FU ORGAN FUNCTION IN THE PULSES

The Fu organs are seen as the Yang aspect, or extensions of the Zang organs, and are used to augment the Yang functions of the Zang organs. The Fu organs provide movement for the Zang organs and have the capacity to bring pathology out of latency, that is, suppressed pathology originating in trauma and the suppression of the personality. For example, Large Intestine points bring out pathology of the Lungs' metal quality or even personality traits pertaining to the Lungs. The Small Intestine and Triple Heater move pathology in the Heart and Pericardium and bring out fire qualities in the personality. The Heart spreads its Qi but is loathe to do so in the presence of Yin factors such as Damp and Cold, but the Small Intestine can dissipate Cold, Wind, Damp and Clear Heat; it deals with climatic factors.

Reading the Fu Organs
To Read the Fu Organs:
  1. Press all three fingers to the moderate level.
  2. Focus on one pulse position while maintaining pressure in the moderate level on the other two positions.

3. Decide whether the sensation you are feeling pertains to the Yang-Fu organ or the Yin-Zang organ. This is done by considering the major functions of the Zang and the Fu organs and locating the corresponding quality or lack thereof in the pulse. Most of the Fu organs do not have many major roles and so this is not nearly as complex as the reading of the Zang organs.

Note: The function of the Fu organs is to move, to discharge, to dissipate (break up) and to release and drain pathologies of their Zang partner. They perform the Yang functions of the pulse position. Therefore rapid pulses in the deep level are pertaining to the Fu organ of that position. This is telling us that the Fu organ is trying to move the pathology contained in the Zang organ of that position.

4. If the quality that pertains to the Fu organs which is found at the moderate level seems to be mirrored in the superficial level or if it seems to extend into the superficial level as a continuous sensation, we can say that we are feeling the Fu organ. Also if a quality pertaining to the Fu organ is found on the deep level and is extending up to the superficial level, we can say the Fu organ is being felt and also that it is very active.

For example, the Large Intestine dissipates Wind and clears Heat. LU-10 can clear Heat, but the Large Intestine can clear Heat more efficiently because the Yang Channels have a greater capacity for moving things out. (Yin has, by contrast of course, a greater capacity to store.) A rapid pulse felt in the deep or moderate level of the Lung pulse that extends up to the superficial level is showing you that the Heat contained in the Lung organ at the deep level is being moved out to the exterior via the Large Intestine.

The Bladder organ can be felt at the cusp of the Ying and Yuan levels, at about 12 beans of pressure.

ASCENSION OF THE STOMACH (ADVANCED)

This ascension is discernible as a resistance in the pulse between 9 and 12 beans of pressure in the right guan position. The Stomach's main function is to descend Qi. It moves food and Gu Qi down the digestive tract and connects with its Yang Ming partner the Large Intestine. But there is also an ascending component to the Stomach, as another of its major functions is the provision of Jin-Thin Fluids, which are ascended via Chong Mai from ST-42 to the sensory orifices. It is the Stomach that provides the mediumship that allows us to have a "lens" to perceive the world. This includes the fluids for perception in the sinuses, the nasal cavity, the taste buds and the aural cavities. If this fluid is not ascended effectively everything looks lackluster or polluted; nothing seems exciting. This elevation goes through the Heart since Chong is involved and so the Heart is also elevated. This is how we are able to perceive beauty. The capacity of the Heart to be excited or enthusiastic about life depends on the capacity of the Stomach to ascend its Pure Yang (pure Jin-Thin fluids).

Earlier we saw that the general descension of Stomach Qi is felt as a strengthening of the pulse as you push from the superficial to the moderate level. We also saw that the ascension of the Spleen is felt as a resistance as you continue pressing through the moderate level and into the deep level. In very advanced pulse taking, the ascending function of the Stomach is felt in the first part of that continued pressing, that is, the first part of the resistance which would be between 9 and 12 beans of pressure. Beyond (deeper than) 12 beans you are feeling purely the ascending function of the Spleen.

FREQUENTLY ASKED QUESTION
If the Yin organs are felt at the deep level of the pulse, how can it be that we are detecting Yang organ function at the deep level?
The Yang organs function as extensions of the Yin organs to move pathology away from the Yin organs. If a rapid quality is felt at the deep level and that quality extends upward in the pulse to the moderate or superficial level, it is telling us that the Yang organ is functioning in its capacity to clear pathology from that Yin organ.

CHAPTER 4

DIRECTIONAL PULSES AND ORGAN COMMUNICATION

Note: See the preface to Chapters 3 and 4 on page 59. before commencing this chapter.

HISTORICAL ROOTS OF DIRECTIONAL PULSES

Directional pulses are a feature of Chapter 11, Scroll 5 of Wang Shu He's second century CE text, the *Mai Jing* (The Pulse Classic). In this book appear the practices of the most prominent practitioners in the Han Dynasty: Hua To and Zhang Zhong Jing (who, incidentally, were competitors) and Bian Que. By the time of the Song Dynasty, directional pulses had disappeared and only static pulses remained. This is partly because the complement channels—the Sinew, Luo, Divergent and Eight Extraordinary Channels—had gone into disuse by that time. Hence, Li Shi Zhen's famous pulse book describes only static pulses, 27 in all.

The practice of directional pulses was not lost, however, from the time of the *Mai Jing*. These teachings, no doubt in somewhat varying forms, were preserved in oral lineages often protected by rules of discipleship. The way in which these pulses were practiced has been in the hands of a rare few individuals since the Song Dynasty, and so this chapter comprises perhaps the most treasured information I am sharing in this volume. It is certainly the information I am most excited about and find invaluable every hour in my clinic. I hope that it will profoundly expand your pulse inquiries.

STATIC AND DIRECTIONAL PULSES

Static pulse taking is very widely used and can provide essential information. Specifically, static pulses tell us the status and quantities of Qi and mediumship. They are single, focused inquiries and are read without moving the finger. The pulse is read at any of the positions and any of the three general depths. Observations about its quality and rate are made, but no inquiry is made about the behavior of that pulse in response to the movement of the practitioner's finger.

Directional pulses, by contrast, involve the practitioner's generation of hydraulic actions in the radial artery. These movements involve one, two or three fingers, and resemble a pumping action. Both static and directional pulses are important, but directional pulses readily provide information regarding communication between organs. Static pulses, read without moving the finger, tell us the status and quantities of Qi and mediumship. If we only have information from static pulses, we need to rely on other diagnostics or intuition because static pulses do not tell us where the pathology is coming from or where it is going. It is likely that we can't even be sure where the pathology is. This is because compromised functioning of a channel or an organ can create effects in another channel or organ. In static pulse taking, when the finger depresses a pulse that pulse position is isolated; it is not communicating with its neighboring organ. Therefore one is not able to see the dynamic exchange between two or more pulses—the dynamic conversation between organs. In static pulses we are also unable to see the dynamic movements between the various depths of the pulse, since each depth is inquired about separately, if at all.

THE IMPORTANCE OF DIRECTIONAL PULSES

Directional pulses are derived from the basic concept that function creates form. In Chinese medicine perhaps the clearest manifestation of this idea occurs in the musculoskeletal system; the way in which we use our body causes it to form in a certain way. For example, the skeletal structure of an obese person has to shift and change to accommodate a weight distribution for which it was not built. A heavy backpack worn habitually only on one shoulder can cause that shoulder to shift and become lower than the other; the function required of the shoulder has affected the actual structure of the shoulder. Similarly, the way in which an organ is performing creates the shape of the pulse. Movements of the finger enable us to read the shape of the pulse in order to see the function (the action) that created the (static) form.

Directional pulses tell us whether there is a problem with the actual organ or whether the pathology is resulting from a failure of communication between organs. If a "directional" action of the finger in one position fails to produce a response in another position, we can deduce that the pathology is in the organ itself, not the channel. If you cannot generate communication between two given pulses using the actions of your fingers, or if you can't create communication in the pulses using spoken dialogue with the patient, there exists an actual visceral organ problem. For example, if the pulse is rapid at a deep level and you can't change it with palpation of the pulses or dialogue with the patient as you are taking the pulses, it's likely there is Heat in the organ itself.

Directional pulses are invaluable in determining the class of channel to be treated and then the exact channel within that class. They also tell us which medium needs to be tended in order for a treatment to be successful. In directional pulses, changes within the position and changes between positions are noted. If the guan position is released, perhaps the cun changes, perhaps the chi changes. These changes reflect the quality of communication between the organs. The early masters were particularly interested in these observations.

Directional pulses reveal the location of excesses and deficiencies. Wherever there is an excess there will be a deficiency and vice versa. We can see whether a wiry or a tight pulse is present due to a pathogenic factor (cold) or whether the tightness is a healthy reaction of the body as it rectifies the lack of something, such as the deficiency of a humor. This kind of information is crucially important since the correct treatments for either possibility are virtually polar opposites of each other. In the first case we would be scattering cold, but in the second case we would be aggressively nourishing the deficient medium—two very different treatments for different causes of a tight or wiry pulse. To unblock an accumulation (tightness) if it is present due to a deficiency would result in the loss of more mediumship and a worsening of the condition. The information gleaned in these pulses can be the difference between a treatment that is a complete success and one that is way off the mark.

ORGAN FUNCTION IN DIRECTIONAL PULSES

THE BREADTH OF INQUIRY

The following list describes the inquiries made in the examination of Directional Pulses.

1. Are the Lungs capable of Dispersing?
2. Does Spleen Qi ascend to the Lungs?
3. Is Triple Heater expressing something from the Jing?
4. Is Kidney Yang escaping?
5. Does Stomach Qi descend to the intestines?
6. Does Lung Qi descend to the Kidneys to nourish postnatal Qi?
7. Does Lung Yin descend to the Lower Jiao?
8. Does Kidney Yang finance Wei Qi to enable the Lungs to perform their dispersing function?
9. Does Heart Qi disperse?
10. Do Liver Qi and Liver Blood ascend to engender Heart Qi and Heart Blood?
11. Does Liver Blood Descend to the Kidneys to nourish Kidney Yin?
12. Does the Heart communicate to the Kidneys?
13. Do the Kidneys communicate to the Heart?

THE IMPORTANCE OF THE ABOVE FINDINGS:

1. *The Lungs disperse Qi.*

   This function enables the Lungs to expel External Pathogenic Factors (EPFs). It is a measure of the readiness and effectiveness of the immune system.

2. *Spleen Qi finances Lung Qi by ascending its Qi to the Lungs.*

   The Spleen ascends its Qi to support Lung Qi. Lung Qi is determined by the adequacy of the connection between the Middle Jiao and the Lungs.

3. *Triple Heater moves pathology out of the Jing.*

   Triple Heater moves pathology from the Yuan level out to the Wei level for elimination.

4. *Stomach Qi descends to the intestines.*

   The downward motion of intestinal function comes from the Stomach.

5. *Lung Qi descends to the Kidneys.*

   The Lungs descend Qi to the Kidneys. This action provides part of the postnatal replenishment of Kidney Qi.

6. *Lung Yin descends to the Lower Jiao.*

   The Lungs descend Yin to the Lower Jiao to moisten the Large Intestine.

7. **The Lungs gather reinforcements of Yang Qi from the Kidneys.**

   The Kidneys grasp Lung Qi. Yang Qi is engendered at the chi position of the right hand and manifests at the cun position of the right hand. That is to say that the Kidneys support Lung Qi. And Kidney Yang is the origin of Wei Qi. If Wei Qi (which is controlled by the Lungs) is not able to deal with a pathogenic factor, Wei Qi then retreats to the chest where the Lungs (and Zhong Qi) reorientate to the bowels to cause urination and defecation of the pathogen. During this process, the Lungs descend to the Kidneys either to recycle Wei Qi (returning it to Kidney Yang which is on the right side) or the Lungs descend to the Kidneys to gather more Wei Qi, to reinforce Lung Qi. (Interestingly this language originates from the end of the Warring States period and the Western Jin period when reinforcements were needed in warfare.) The Lungs, like an emissary, communicate with the Kidneys to obtain reinforcements and then ascend with those reinforcements in hand. We need to make sure the Lungs are able to access the Yang Qi. This is seen at the deep level of the chi position.

8. *The Heart disperses Qi.*

   The Heart's main function is to shine its great light outward.

9. *Liver Qi and Liver Blood ascend to engender Heart Qi and Heart Blood.*

   Heart Blood and Qi are derived from Liver Blood.

10. *Liver Blood descends to the Kidneys to nourish Kidney Yin.*

    Liver Blood is a postnatal origin of Kidney Yin.

11. **The Heart communicates to the Kidneys.**

    The Heart shines its light to the Kidneys, bringing illumination and self-reflection to the unknown.

12. *The Kidneys communicate to the Heart.*

The Kidneys reveal the curriculum of life to the Heart which in turn meets the inherent challenges with its beam of shining light.

DIRECTIONAL PULSE TAKING METHOD

At first, this chapter will seem complicated. It's not, really. I've included as many diagrams as possible. Fortunately, once you grasp the movement of Spleen Qi to the Lungs you have the main building block for the whole system. The rest of the process is merely duplicating the same action in different positions. After a short while it becomes easy to perform the actions. I'm sure you will find the result quite remarkable and its addition to your practice invaluable.

POSITIONING THE FINGERS FOR DIRECTIONAL PULSE TAKING

Pulse Neutral Position

The starting position for directional pulse taking is a position I call Pulse Neutral. The fingers in the cun and guan positions sit at 9 beans of pressure (squarely in the moderate level of the pulse) and the finger at the chi position is at 12 beans of pressure (at the interface of Ying and Yuan Qi).

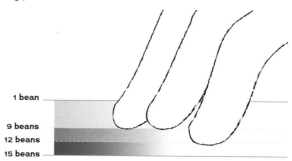

The Tilt and Release Actions

Directional pulses measure vectors, that is, the direction in which mediumship and Qi are moving. Directional pulses involve two types of action: the tilt and the release.

The Tilt Action and the Pop

The tilt action is a compound movement made by two fingers. At the same time that one finger is moving down (toward the bone) another finger is moving up (away from the bone). The resulting hydraulic action in the artery causes an accent on the pulse at the finger being lifted. I call this the "pop". The pop is a surge of energy. The pop affects one single beat of the pulse.

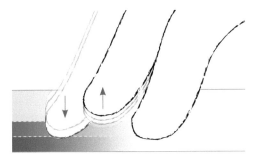

The finger action in the tilt is extremely tiny. Often, when I teach this technique, students say at first that they cannot see or feel the action of my fingers on their wrist. After a few minutes, their attention is honed and they can feel it. It's just a matter of focus, of finely tuned attention.

To practice the action away from the pulse, however, use gross actions, just to get orientated. The resting position for the tilt action is 9 beans in the cun and guan, and 12 beans in the chi position.

The range of motion in the tilt is about three beans in either direction. The cun and guan fingers are at times going to move up toward 6 beans of pressure or down toward 12 beans of pressure.

The chi finger will at times move down toward 15 beans and sometimes up toward 9 beans of pressure.

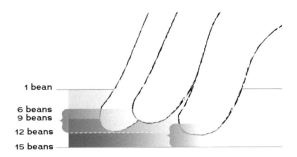

With practice, these actions become smaller and smaller and the readings can be done with movements of three beans or fewer, up or down.

The Release Action

The release action tests for floating pulses. To practice it, go to 12 beans at the right cun position. Very, very slowly release your pressure. Allow the journey from nine beans to one bean to take about 30 seconds. Some pulses reveal pathology when they float. Others reveal pathology when they do not float. When focusing on a pulse that should float, I write down the degree to which a pulse is in fact floating, based on how far it comes up. For example, if the Lung pulse floats from nine beans to one bean, I'll write "100%" on the chart. If it floats up to six beans and then is lost under the fingers, I'll write "30%" on the chart.

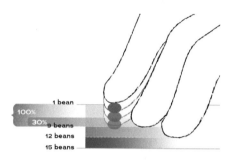

THE SEQUENCE OF DIRECTIONAL PULSES

Note: Directional pulses are just one part of a full pulse diagnosis. See chapter 6 for fully comprehensive step by step protocols.

1. Assume pulse neutral position.

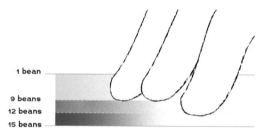

2. Release: Are the Lungs capable of Dispersing their Qi to maintain the distribution of Wei Qi? As slowly as possible release pressure from the Lung pulse and allow your finger to follow the pulse upward toward the skin. The pulse should follow your finger all the way up to skin level—to one bean—and may scatter at that point.

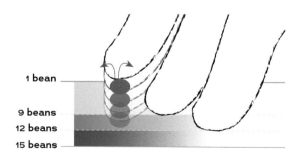

a. If the Lung pulse does follow your finger all the way to the surface, we can say that the Lungs are fully dispersing Qi.

b. If the Lung pulse does not follow your finger all the way to the surface, we can say that the Lungs are not fully dispersing Qi. If you are going very slowly and yet lose the pulse under your finger at, for example, the half way mark, you could say the Lungs are dispersing to about 50% of capacity.

3. Tilt: Does Spleen Qi ascend to the Lungs, to finance Lung Qi? Simultaneously press both the Spleen and Kidney pulses down the tiniest amount and at the same time release the tiniest amount of pressure from the Lung pulse. The Lung pulse should give one pop during the next beat.

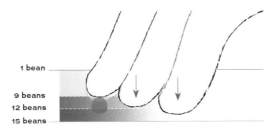

a. If the Lung pulse does pop, we can say that Spleen Qi does ascend to the Lungs.

b. If the Lung pulse does not pop, we can say that Spleen Qi does not ascend to the Lungs.

4. Release: Is Triple Heater expressing something from the Jing? Is Kidney Yang escaping? As slowly as possible, release pressure from the Kidney Yang pulse (right chi) and allow your finger to follow the pulse upward toward the skin. The pulse should stop following the finger while still within the Yuan level. If it stays in contact with your finger as you lift it, keep going and note the point at which it stops following the finger.

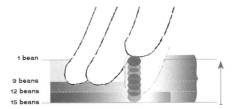

a. If the pulse is lost within the moderate level, we can say there is imbalance in the Pericardium and its facilitation of the communication of Heart and Kidneys.

b. If the pulse comes up to the Wei level, we can say that Kidney Yang is escaping.

c. If the pulse comes up to the top of the Wei level and is very rapid, we can say that the Triple Heater mechanism is engaged in trying to eradicate pathology from the Yuan level.

5. Tilt: Does Stomach Qi descend to the intestines? From the neutral position, press the Spleen pulse down the tiniest amount and at the same time, release the tiniest amount of pressure from the Kidney pulse. The Kidney pulse should give one pop during the next beat.

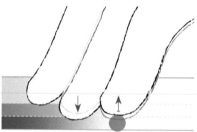

a. If the Kidney pulse does pop we can say that Stomach Qi does descend.

b. If the Kidney pulse does not pop, we can say that the Stomach is not descending or not descending optimally.

c. If the Stomach is not descending and the vector from Spleen to Lungs seems overly pronounced, the Stomach might be ascending; you may be finding rebellious Stomach Qi. To find out if this is the case, raise your cun and guan fingers a few beans and check the guan position to cun position vector at a more superficial level. If it still pronounced, there is rebellious Qi of the Stomach.

6. Tilt: Do Lung Qi and Lung Yin descend to the Kidneys to enable the Kidneys to produce Kidney Qi and to moisten the Large Intestine? Simultaneously press the Lung and Spleen pulses down the tiniest amount and at the same time, release the tiniest amount of pressure from the Kidney pulse. The Kidney pulse should pop during the next beat.

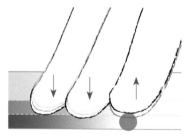

a. If the Kidney pulse does pop we can say that Lung Qi does descend and is grasped by the Kidneys.

b. If the Kidney pulse does not pop, we can say that the Lungs are not descending or that they are not descending optimally. A weakness in Kidney Yang could then be a false weakness (appearing to be weak when the Kidneys are not weak) since the Lungs are not nourishing the Kidneys.

c. Note: You might feel that the Lung Qi descends under your fingers but not all the way to the Kidneys. The Kidneys are not popping because the Lung Qi is not reaching all the way to the Kidneys. Classically, Kidneys grasping Lung Qi implied the complete descension of Lung Qi. In other words, if the descension of Lung Qi was complete, the Kidneys automatically received that Qi.

Note: The Stomach serves as an emissary for this action. If this vector is absent, it may mean that there is a blockage in the Middle Jiao.

7. Tilt (Advanced): Does Kidney Yang finance Wei Qi (at the Lung position) to enable the Lungs to perform their dispersing function? Press the Kidney pulse down the tiniest amount and almost immediately after that, press the Spleen pulse down the tiniest amount and almost immediately after that, release the tiniest amount of pressure from the Lungs. The second pressure (the one at the Spleen) should palpably increase the hydraulic pressure moving up to the Lungs. The Lung pulse should give one pop during the next beat.

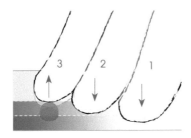

a. If the Lung pulse does pop we can say that Kidney Yang does finance Wei Qi.

b. During this advanced compound tilt you might notice a connection moving upward from the Kidney pulse to the Spleen pulse. Kidney Yang is supporting Spleen Yang. This leg of the pulse reflects the third trajectory of the Kidney Primary Channel which connects KI-2 to SP-8 and is the basis of digestive Qi.

8. Release: Does Heart Qi Disperse? Now, on the left wrist, much should be familiar already. As slowly as possible release pressure from the Heart pulse and allow your finger to follow the pulse upward toward the skin. The pulse should follow your finger much of the way to the skin level, and then scatter.

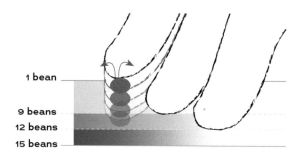

1 bean

9 beans

12 beans

15 beans

a. If the Heart pulse does follow your finger into the Wei level, we can say that the Heart is dispersing Qi.

b. If the Heart pulse does not follow your finger all the way to the surface, we can say that the Heart is not fully dispersing Qi.

9. Tilt: Do Liver Qi and Liver Blood ascend to engender Heart Qi and Heart Blood?
Press the Liver pulse down the tiniest amount and at the same time, release the tiniest amount of pressure from the Heart pulse. The Heart pulse should give a pop during the next beat.

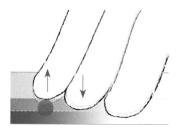

a. If the Heart pulse does pop we can say that Liver Blood does ascend to the Heart.

b. If the Heart pulse does not pop, we can say that the Liver is not ascending or that it is not ascending optimally.

10. Tilt: Does Liver Blood Descend to the Kidneys to nourish Kidney Yin?
Press the Liver pulse down the tiniest amount and at the same time, release the tiniest amount of pressure from the Kidney pulse. The Kidney pulse should give a pop during the next beat.

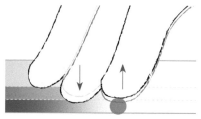

a. If the Kidney pulse does pop we can say that Liver Blood does nourish Kidney Yin.

b. If the Kidney pulse does not pop, we can say that Liver Blood is not descending to the Kidneys or that it is not descending optimally.

11. Tilt: (Advanced) Does the Heart communicate to the Kidneys?

Press the Heart position and, almost immediately after that, press the Liver position down the tiniest amount, and almost immediately after that release the tiniest amount of pressure from the Kidney pulse. The Kidney pulse should give a pop during the next beat.

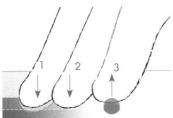

a. If the Kidney pulse does pop we can say that the Heart does communicate to the Kidneys.

b. If the Kidney pulse does not pop, we can say the communication of the Heart to the Kidneys is impeded somehow.

Note: The Liver serves as the emissary for this action. This means that in order for this communication to happen, the diaphragm must be free. A blockage in the Heart-Kidney vector may indicate a diaphragmatic blockage.

12. Tilt: Do the Kidneys communicate to the Heart? As the Kidneys contain Ancestral Qi—the repository of a person's destiny—and the Heart contains the individual's current experience of identity, reading the communication of Kidney to Heart essentially explores how well an individual is living his or her destiny. Traditionally, this pulse reading is considered to be intruding on the individual's sovereignty and is left unexplored, unread. This is beyond the role of the clinician/patient or even master/student relationship. The technique for reading this pulse, however, is no different from the others and is hypothetically explained here. Press the Kidney pulse down the tiniest amount and at the same time, release the tiniest amount of pressure from the Heart pulse. The Heart pulse should give one pop during the next beat.

a. If the Heart pulse does pop we can say that the Kidneys do communicate to the Heart.

93

b. If the Heart pulse does not pop, we can say the communication of the Kidneys to the Heart is impeded somehow.

SUMMARY OF DIRECTIONAL PULSE TAKING

Pressure must be maintained in all positions at all times.

1. *Assume pulse neutral position.*
2. **Release:** Are the Lungs capable of Dispersing? Release the Lung pulse.
3. **Tilt:** Does Spleen Qi ascend to the Lungs? Press both the Spleen and Kidney pulses down and release pressure from the Lung pulse.
4. **Release:** Is Triple Heater expressing something from the Jing? Is Kidney Yang escaping? Release pressure from the Kidney Yang pulse.
5. **Tilt:** Does Stomach Qi descend to the intestines? Press the Spleen pulse down and release the Kidney pulse.
6. **Tilt:** Do Lung Qi and Lung Yin descend to the Kidneys to enable the Kidneys to produce Kidney Yang and Kidney Yin? Press the Lung and Spleen pulses down the tiniest amount and release the Kidney pulse.
7. **Tilt:** (Advanced) Does Kidney Yang finance Wei Qi (at the Lung position) to enable the Lungs to perform their dispersing function? Press the Kidney pulse down, then press the Spleen pulse down, then release pressure from the Lungs.
8. **Release:** Does Heart Qi Disperse? Release pressure from the Heart pulse.
9. **Tilt:** Do Liver Qi and Liver Blood ascend to engender Heart Qi and Heart Blood? Press the Liver pulse down and release pressure from the Heart pulse.
10. **Tilt:** Does Liver Blood Descend to the Kidneys to nourish Kidney Yin? Press the Liver pulse down and release pressure from the Kidney pulse.
11. **Tilt:** (Advanced) Does the Heart communicate to the Kidneys? Press the Heart pulse down, then the Liver position down, then release pressure from the Kidney pulse.
12. **Tilt:** Do the Kidneys communicate to the Heart? (If you choose to look.) Press the Kidney pulse down, then release the tiniest amount of pressure from the Heart pulse.

R   L

superficial
moderate   LU   HT   superficial
deep   moderate
                                deep

superficial
moderate   SP   LR   superficial
deep   moderate
                                deep

superficial
moderate   KI Yang   KI Yin   superficial
deep   moderate
                                deep

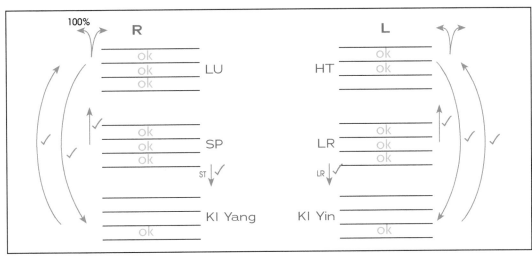

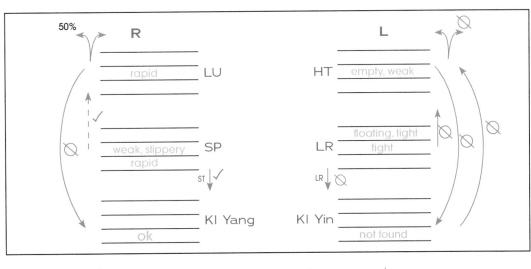

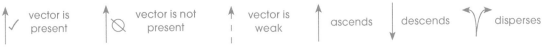

vector is present   vector is not present   vector is weak   ascends   descends   disperses

VERY BASIC TREATMENT OF DIRECTIONAL PULSE FINDINGS

Learning acupuncture is a long process in which acupuncture school is but a foundation. Point energetics are learned, then learned again, then learned in layers of historical meaning. Although points have function independently, point directionality and function are strongest in the context of a well-designed treatment. For example, BL-40 is sometimes taught as having the function of easing back pain, but that function is by far stronger and clearer when used in the context of a Bladder Divergent treatment. The acupuncturist gradually builds a personal knowledge of interwoven functionality of point energetics and associations.

AN EXAMPLE:

A patient complained of cough. The pulses show the Lungs were strong but that there was rebellious Stomach Qi. The Lungs were expressing the rebellion of the Stomach. A point that descends Lung Qi would not provide successful treatment. The treatment strategy must include descending the Stomach. There are many points that descend the Stomach, for example, ST-5 or ST-30. In this case CV-12 might best be chosen to perform this function since it is also the first point on the Lung Primary Channel.

Note: The list below comprises basic teaching examples only. There are countless ways to correct and generate these vectors using knowledge of point function. The correct approach will vary from patient to patient according to their strengths and weaknesses and their accompanying signs and symptoms.

1. *Lung dispersal.* To disperse the Lungs, choose a point with that function. For example, LU-1, LU-7 or LU-8 disperse the Lungs.

2. *Spleen to Lung ascension.* KI-2, SP-8, and LU-1 together ascend Spleen Qi to the Lungs.

3. *Kidney Yang is escaping or Triple Heater releases toxins.* Nourishing Yin enables Yang to be anchored. Bleeding GB-36 releases toxicity from the Yuan level. (If practicing the Complement Channels, Triple Heater Divergent Channel needled deep-superficial-deep returns toxicity to the Yuan level for later expulsion.)

4. *Stomach descension.* ST-5, CV-12 and ST-30 descend the Stomach, for example.

5. *Lung Qi and Lung Yin descension to the Kidneys.* Choose a point that descends Lung Qi, for example, LU-5. Connecting the water point of the Lungs and the metal point of the Kidneys would be one way to create this descension.

6. *Kidney Yang generating Wei Qi.* Usually ascension of Kidney Yang generates stimulation of this vector as long as blockages are not in play. KI-2 to SP-8 ascends Kidney Yang to the Spleen and LU-1 takes it up to the Lungs. See Inter-Jiao Blockages, page 97.

7. *Liver ascension to Heart.* I usually use a whole channel to create this vector, such as Yin Wei Mai or Liver Divergent, but as points, LR-14 and CV-14 needled with intention to connect, create this vector. The second branch of the Liver Primary Channel also makes

this vector: LR-14, CV-12, PC-1.

8. *Heart dispersal.* This vector seems only to appear if the patient feels connection to humanity or if the person has optimism, which perhaps only exist in parallel. The practitioner's optimism and open heart create this vector.

9. *Liver descension.* LR-14 can produce this vector. Yin Wei Mai produces this vector.

10. *Heart to Kidney communication and Kidney to Heart communication.* I usually use whole channels such as Chong or Yin Wei Mai to create these vectors. KI-21 creates these vectors on its own, however.

INTER-JIAO BLOCKAGES: THE DIAPHRAGM AND DAI MAI

Inter-Jiao blockages can prevent the free flow of Qi from one organ to another. The most common external cause of these blockages is Cold. Emotions are the most common internal cause. A lack of love results in Cold. Ultimately, if untreated, blockages affect the entire system as the movement of Qi is progressively impeded. Blockages can prevent the success of any treatment and must be released. Fortunately, the technique of Directional pulses enables the practitioner to find blockages relatively easily.

Inter-Jiao blockages should not be confused with tightness. Very often, tight pulses indicate a positive response in the body to a lack of some kind of mediumship (Fluids, Blood, Yin). For example, if the Liver pulse is tight, it's likely that there is a Blood deficiency and the body is trying to hold onto Blood. Releasing this tightness can result in prolonging the Blood deficiency as the body gathers more Qi to reinstate the tightness in order to place Blood in reserve. It's essential to separate pathological tightness from tightness generated by the body as a response to pathology. Tightness generated as a response to pathology is not pathology itself. In the case above, the nourishment of Blood would result in the Liver relaxing. That is, the tight response to the pathology of Blood deficiency falls away when Blood deficiency is resolved.

Inter-Jiao blockages can cause an organ to appear deficient when it is not. For example, the Lungs might appear weak, but that may be an illusion; they may simply not be receiving Qi from the Spleen because the diaphragm is blocking it. (Qi from a weak or tight Spleen might not reach the Lungs either.) Tonifying Lung Qi would not yield lasting results, or no result at all, but if the lack of communication is due to a blockage of the diaphragm, releasing that blockage in the diaphragm would enable the Lungs to act in their full capacity. The Lungs could also appear weak if Kidney Yang is not reaching the Spleen. This could show as tightness in Kidney Yang, a Yang deficiency, a blockage in the low back, or a blockage in Dai Mai. Tonifying Lung Qi or Spleen Qi would yield no positive result in the Lungs, but treating the Kidneys or the blockage in Dai Mai would.

Diaphragmatic blockages are likely present if:
- on both wrists the guan positions do not communicate up to the cun positions.
- while performing any of the described tilt actions to or from the cun position, the position being pressed becomes stronger and the receiving pulse does not react. For example, when checking that the Spleen is able to ascend its Qi to the Lungs (pressing the guan position down and releasing the Lung position) the Spleen pulse surges but the Lung pulse does not respond at all, a blockage is present in the diaphragm.
- there is a palpable bulge between the cun and the guan positions.

Dai Mai blockage is likely present if:
- on both wrists the guan positions do not communicate down to the chi positions.
- while performing any of the described tilt actions to or from the chi position, the position being pressed becomes stronger and the receiving pulse does not react. For example, when checking that the Liver is able to descend its Qi to the Kidneys (pressing the guan position down and releasing the Kidney position) the Liver pulse surges but the Kidney pulse does not respond at all, a blockage is present in Dai Mai.
- there is a palpable bulge between the guan and the chi positions.

TREATMENT OF INTER-JIAO BLOCKAGES

There are limitless options for releasing inter-Jiao blockages. Choose points with which you resonate. These are the ones I resonate with in case it's helpful.

To release the diaphragm: release LR-14. Insert very obliquely, reduce strongly and remove. Or release LR-13 in a similar way. Or reduce LR-6 and LU-6. Or reduce BL-17 at the Hua To position.

To release Dai Mai, needle GB-41, GB-26, GB-27 and GB-28 unilaterally (left in males, right in females) and vibrate until the patient feels a very subtle descending feeling in the lower abdomen.
To further release blockages, consider releasing a tight pulse by reducing the Mu point of the related organ.

It is, of course, essential to release any Sinew pulse (any tight, superficial pulse). See page 102 for a full discussion. The method chosen could involve sliding cups or gua sha on the Sinew Channel indicated, a full Sinew treatment, or the release of the Jing-Well point of the channel indicated. Most of these releases take a few minutes.

Check the pulses to ensure the blockage has been released before proceeding with the remainder of the treatment. If the blockage has been cleared:

- either or both of the guan positions will freely communicate up to the cun or down to the chi.
- a pulse will not become fuller when it is pressed during a tilt action.
- bulges between the guan and either the cun or chi will no longer be present.

REFUSAL

Refusal in the pulses means the healthy circulation of Qi is interrupted not by deficiency nor by blockage, but because the receiving organ for some reason is not receptive to the Qi that nourishes it. The possibility of a blockage should be eliminated before considering refusal. The tendency of an organ to refuse Qi or mediumship can be determined while taking directional pulses. For example, while using the Tilt action to determine whether the Lungs are able to receive Qi from the Spleen, if you find that the Spleen pulse becomes fuller (instead of the Lung pulse, which we would expect) the Lungs are said to be refusing Spleen Qi. The organ refusing Qi can do so in order to protect an emotional status quo. For example, the Lungs can refuse Qi if there is a conscious or unconscious desire to suppress grief. The added Qi would perhaps stimulate the Lungs to express the grief, but the patient is not ready or unwilling to process it.

REFUSAL IN THE KIDNEY YANG POSITION

If the Kidneys refuse blood from the Heart it is said that the Pericardium is preventing Heart-Kidney communication. This is confirmed by examining both wrists at the same time. A pulse will emerge in the moderate level of the Kidney Yang position and there can be a tightening at the Heart position at the same time. If, conversely, the Heart refuses Blood the patient is not ready to look at emotional issues. This, of course, should be respected.

FAILURE TO RECEIVE

Failure to receive is also determined during directional pulse taking. If, while using the Tilt action, Qi or Fluid is felt moving toward the receiving organ but the receiving organ does not accept it, the receiving organ is said to fail to receive. This is sometimes felt while determining communication between Lungs and Kidneys when Qi is felt leaving the Lung position but does not cause a reaction (pop) in the Kidney position. In this case, the Lungs are descending Qi but the Kidneys are not receiving (grasping) it. An organ might not receive Qi if it is lacking the Yang Qi to hold the incoming medium in place. It might also not receive Qi in order to maintain a convenient emotional status quo. For example, in patients who are reluctant to enter into what they feel is their true path, the Heart might not receive communication from the Kidneys because to do so would raise awareness of their destiny and the responsibility to live it. If the Heart doesn't receive Blood, recommend the patient stop all hot spices, garlic and coffee; the Heart may be occupied scattering Heat.

REFUSAL VERSUS FAILURE TO RECEIVE

Refusal and failure to receive differ in that during refusal the destination organ pushes the delivery back at the organ of origin (the sender), causing pulse of the organ of origin to swell momentarily. Failure to receive implies the receiving organ would be happy to accept delivery if it had the means to hold onto it.

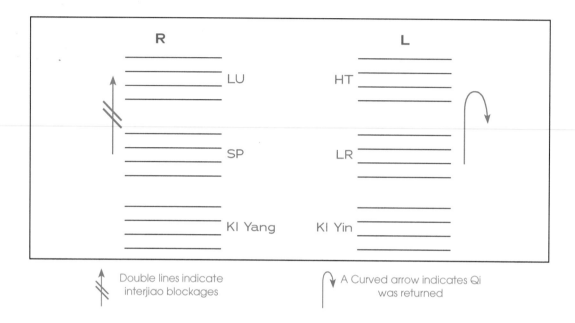

Double lines indicate interjiao blockages

A Curved arrow indicates Qi was returned

CHAPTER 5

PULSES OF THE CHANNELS OF ACUPUNCTURE

This chapter includes pulses for the Primary Channels as well as pulses for the Sinew, Luo, Divergent and Eight Extraordinary Channels, the four classes of channel collectively known as the Complement Channels. The Complement Channels comprise the bulk of the complete system of acupuncture. While the Primary Channels are responsible for minute-to-minute functioning, the role of the Complement Channels is quite different. They are responsible for dealing with pathology that the body has not been able to clear and to keep pathology away from the organs where it could lead to serious and life-threatening illness. The Complement Channels are present to preserve life, to preserve humanity.

The Complement Channels and their functions are introduced in the earliest Classics of Chinese Medicine. Their detailed functions and treatment protocols were extraordinarily developed from that time and through the Tang Dynasty (618-907, CE). This knowledge was held and transmitted in an extensive and precise oral tradition. Between the beginning of the Song Dynasty (960-1279 CE) and the late twentieth century, these channels were not in common use. Indeed, their pulses do not appear in post-Song writings.

The Complement Channels have their own particular pulse diagnosis techniques. I still find it quite remarkable that when you ask the pulses for specific information in any channel category they will immediately oblige. By this I mean that if you have decided before making contact with the pulse that you would like to investigate the Eight Extraordinary Channels, the pulses will present Eight Extraordinary information more emphatically than other information. This is a result of the intention of the practitioner.

It should be noted, however, that if there is a sinew issue, it can show in the pulses even as we have our attention on another level of inquiry. This is telling us that we must release blockages in the exterior before deeper work can begin. Usually that requires a short sinew treatment to begin the session or a little time with gua sha or cupping, after which the selected treatment can go ahead.

Below you will find two contrasting methods, each for Sinew and Divergent pulses. They appear contradictory to one another but the pulses react according to your method. This is why there is no correct pulse taking method and why we have seen the emergence of a myriad of pulse taking styles, many of which are completely workable. In any method the intention of the practitioner is crucially important. If the inquiry is conducted with a clear intention and clear method, the pulses will in turn deliver a clear message.

As we'd expect, the pulse of each channel category is reflected at its level of Qi.

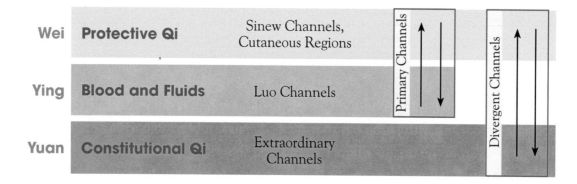

Note: For detailed information about pathology of the Complement Channels and the use of these channels therapeutically, please refer to my book, *Advanced Acupuncture, A Clinic Manual*: Protocols for the Complement Channels (2013).

SINEW CHANNEL PULSES

The Sinew Channels are the simplest to diagnose in all of pulse taking. Since the function of the Sinew Channels is to conduct Wei Qi to defend or shield the exterior, pathology of the Sinew Channels is reflected in tightness at the Wei level of the pulse. Tightness results when Wei Qi is in the act of defense. The sinew is tightening to defend against further invasion of a pathogen and/or the sinew is tight as it tries to expel a pathogen. The tightness is easily felt at between one and six beans of pressure depending on the sinew implicated. The pulse in question can feel as though it is guarding against your finger somewhere in the superficial level, almost pushing the finger away.

Tight pulses in the Wei level (between one and six beans of pressure) indicate that the exterior (a Sinew Channel) must be released by gua sha, cupping, or with a Sinew treatment.

	CUN	GUAN	CHI
1-3 Beans of pressure	Tai Yang	Shao Yang	Yang Ming
3-6 Beans of Pressure	Tai Yin	Shao Yin	Jue Yin

LEFT VERSUS RIGHT SINEW PULSES

Sinew pulses in the right wrist indicate a mild condition; sinew pulses in the left wrist indicate a more severe condition. This is because the right wrist demonstrates the body's capacity to push the pathogen out while the left wrist demonstrates the body's capacity to make or keep a pathogen latent. A sinew pulse in the right hand shows that the body is in the process of pushing a pathogen out; it just needs a helping hand. A sinew pulse in the left hand means that the body is in the process of sending the pathogen into a state of latency because there are not enough resources to mount an attempt to push it out. For example, a sinew pulse found in the right chi position would indicate a Yang Ming Sinew condition that a simple sinew treatment would resolve, whereas the same pulse in the left chi indicates a severe Yang Ming Sinew condition. If sinew pulses are found in the left wrist, both the arm sinews and the leg sinews related to that position are treated since the condition is worsening.

ZANG FU VERSUS SINEW APPROACH

If you are intending to treat an external pathogenic factor with a Zang Fu approach, examine the right cun position to determine the status of the Lungs, since the Lungs control Wei Qi. If you want to treat an external pathogenic factor (EPF) with a Sinew Channel approach, look for superficial pulses in any position. If a superficial or floating-tight pulse is found, it is imperative—during the same session—to treat the sinews first before moving on to treat the main complaint. This treatment need not take long. To treat anything other than the sinews first can easily invite the pathogen to move deeper into the body, risking the illness becoming severe. This is what has happened if a patient tells you that after a treatment the cold they were hoping to fight off went into their chest and they became quite ill. The Primary Channels were not efficiently equipped to release the pathogenic factor.

THE YIN SINEW PULSES

If the pulses are floating and tight but also tight at six beans of pressure (the interface of the Wei and Ying levels) the Yin Sinew Channels are involved. For example, if the pulse is floating and tight at the guan position and also tight at six beans of pressure in the guan, the Shao Yin sinew and the Shao Yang sinew would be treated, in that order.

The sinews are affected at between three and six beans:
1. The cun position reflects the Tai Yin Sinew which affects the chest.
2. The guan position reflects the Shao Yin Sinew which affects the central axis.
3. The chi position reflects the Jue Yin Sinew which affects the abdomen.

The pulse is floating and tight between one and three beans but is also tight between three and six beans:

1. In the cun position it means that a Tai Yang condition is spreading to Tai Yin.
2. In the guan position it means that a Shao Yang condition is spreading to Shao Yin.
3. In the chi position it means that a Yang Ming condition is spreading to Jue Yin.

SLIPPERY AND RAPID COMPLICATIONS

The emergence of floating, tight and slippery pulses at the cun position indicates that the condition is moving into the Shao Yang zone.

If the pulse at the cun or the guan is floating, tight and rapid, the condition is moving into Yang Ming and is deepening.

If the pulse at the chi position is floating, tight and rapid, the condition is in Yang Ming and is severe.

COLD INVASION OF THE SINEWS

Pathology of the Tai Yang Sinew Channel (including the common cold) is the most common of all conditions. Seventy percent of the *Shang Han Lun* is devoted to Tai Yang pathology because all conditions are seen as the result of its incorrect treatment or lack of treatment.

Yang is engendered from the Kidneys. A portion of that Yang becomes Wei Qi, which is then under the command of the Lungs. In terms of the pulse, Yang is engendered at the chi position and manifests in the cun position. The cun position is the position of the Tai Yang Sinew—the biggest conduit of Wei Qi. Its engagement with an external pathogen shows as a tight cun pulse.

The pulse is tight partly because of the invasion of Cold and the attempt of the Tai Yang Sinew to expel that Cold, but particularly the cun is tight because there is a blockage in the dissemination of Yang to the exterior. Yang is blocked and cannot fully become Wei Qi in the first place. In terms of the pulses, there is a blockage preventing the chi position communicating up to the cun position. In other words, Yang Qi, which at the chi position is still a component of Yuan Qi, is unable to convert to Wei Qi and express itself against the pathogenic factor, a failure which is shown when the cun position is tight and not dispersing. The invasion of Cold is causing the blockage to reveal itself because Yang Qi is clearly shown not to be fighting the pathogen. The blockage in turn, ironically, is trapping the Cold. Treatments can fail if blockages are not released. Blockages are discussed on page 87.

- Tai Yang Sinew pulses indicate tightness trapping Cold.
- Shao Yang Sinew pulses indicate tightness trapping Damp.
- Yang Ming Sinew pulses indicate tightness trapping Heat.

SLOW SINEW PULSES

Slow sinew pulses alter the reflexology of the pulses as the pathology is moving inward. Slow pulses in any position indicate a severe condition as Cold is moving inward. The Yin sinew pairs become affected and the standard sinew progression is no longer in play. If the pulse is floating, tight and slow at between one and three beans of pressure and also tight and slow at between three and six beans of pressure, the condition has become severe and has moved not only into the zonally related Arm Yang Sinews of that pulse position but also into the Leg Yin elemental pair.

If the pulse is floating, tight and slow at between one and three beans of pressure and also tight and slow at between three and six beans of pressure:
1. In the cun position, the condition is moving from the Bladder Sinew Channel into the Small Intestine Sinew Channel and also the Kidney Sinew Channel.
2. In the guan position, the condition is moving from the Gallbladder Sinew Channel into the Triple Heater Sinew Channel and also into the Liver Sinew Channel.
3. In the chi position, the condition is moving from the Stomach Sinew Channel into the Large Intestine Sinew Channel and also into the Spleen Sinew Channel.

The remaining Yin Sinew Channels: Heart, Pericardium and Lung Sinews, become affected upon the deep worsening of the severe conditions above, respectively. A deep Kidney Sinew issue can eventually affect the Heart Sinew Channel, a deep Liver Sinew issue can eventually affect the Pericardium Sinew Channel, and a deep Spleen Sinew issue can eventually affect the Lung Sinew Channel. The transmission of the disease to the Arm Yin Sinew Channels indicates a severe condition.

THE INTERNALIZATION OF PATHOLOGY VIA THE SINEW CHANNELS IN THE PULSES

The presence of Yin Sinew pulses (a tight or wiry quality at between three and six beans of pressure) indicates that pathology of the Yang Sinews is starting to internalize but has not yet achieved access to the interior. The pulses will tell you whether the body is trying to move that pathology out or not.

If the pulses are tight between three and six beans of pressure and tending laterally (felt more laterally than you might expect), pathology of the Yin Sinews is moving to the Yang Sinews. It is moving toward the exterior and the body is healing.

If the pulses are tight between three and six beans of pressure and leaning medially, pathology has progressed to the Yin Sinews and, if not treated, can affect the Zang Fu or be diverted to another channel system altogether, likely the Divergent or Luo Channels.

THE RELEASE OF INTERNAL PATHOLOGY TO THE YIN SINEW CHANNELS IN THE PULSES (ADVANCED)

It is imperative that the body clear pathology from the interior. At the very least, it must move pathology from the interior to the exterior. If it chooses to do this via the Sinew Channels, the Yin Sinew Channels will receive the pathology before the Yang sinews do. It will emerge at the Ying level. At six beans of pressure—the cusp of the Wei and Ying levels—you might feel that although the floating pulse is felt medial to the radial artery it is coming at you obliquely, moving laterally. This is a marker of pathology moving outward from the Ying level to the Wei level where the deepest layer of the Wei level—Yin Sinew Channels—are meeting it, receiving it and readying it for passage to the Yang Sinews that will finally expel it. In short, rolling the fingers from the medial to lateral aspect of the pulses traverses you through the Yuan-Ying-Wei progression of pathology clearing.

But here's the interesting part: if you feel that movement—floating tight pulse at six beans of pressure medial to the radial artery but leaning laterally—in the cun position, the pathology is moving out from Jue Yin. This is because ultimate Yin (Jue Yin) must flip to ultimate Yang (Tai Yang). If in the guan position, the pathology is moving outward from Tai Yin. If in the chi position, pathology is moving outward from Shao Yin. Conversely, if the floating tight pulse is medial to the radial artery but moving inward toward the tendon at the cun position, the pathology is moving into Jue Yin. At the guan position it is moving in to Tai Yin and at the chi position it is moving into Shao Yin.

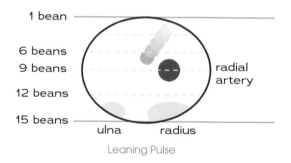

Leaning Pulse

To treat, gua sha the zone diagnosed to assist in the release of the pathogen and free the blood and Qi implicated in the blockage of the Sinew in question. If the surface is released and Ying and Wei are unblocked through gua sha, the pathogen trapped at the Yuan level can emerge and return to the exterior. (Diagnosis requiring Zonal Divergent treatments can be determined this way also, since Divergents release Yuan level pathology to the Wei level. Treat the channel trying to release itself and its zonal pair. For example, if you feel a tight floating pulse at six beans in the chi position, do a Heart and Kidney Zonal Divergent treatment. More on this subject, with details of treatment protocols, is described in *Advanced Acupuncture, A Clinic Manual*.)

SINEW CHANNEL DIAGNOSIS

There are three factors investigated in the process of diagnosing the Sinew Channels.
• Determining which body movement yields the greatest amount of discomfort.
• Observing the location of the pain.
• Noting the location of a sinew pulse.
Each of these examinations may indicate a different channel.

PRIMARY CHANNEL PULSES

Pulse taking for the Primary Channels involves locating blockages in the flow of Blood and Qi. Treatment of the Primary Channels involves releasing these blockages and in so doing, balancing the relationship between interior and exterior, between Yin and Yang. The Primary Channels are conduits of Wei Qi and Ying Qi. Since the aim of their treatment is to balance Wei Qi and Ying Qi, the initial focus in their pulse reading is at the level of six beans of pressure, the juncture of the Wei and Ying levels. This is the point at which the two interact, the shallowest region of the pulse at which Blood and Qi are felt interacting. The Primary Channels also communicate with the organs. Therefore there is an additional focus on 12 beans of pressure where the organs are palpable and the interaction of Blood and Qi is again measurable. At twelve beans, Ying Qi is communicating with the Yuan Qi circulating in the organs. The Primary Channels govern the moment-to-moment functioning of the body by maintaining the connections between Wei, Ying and Yuan Qi. The Primary Channels, while only part of the complete channel system, show the status of Blood and Fluids, and allow treatment of these crucial connections.

The Primary Channels are manufactured by the Zang Fu to act as conduits for messages emanating from the Zang Fu. Regardless of where the Primary Channels originate anatomically, their pulses come from the Zang Fu in the torso.

The pulses are like relay stations for the Zang Fu, transmitting details about Zang Fu activity to the surface (to the pulse). The practitioner deciphers the signal the organ transmits. The relaying of this transmission is the function of the Primary Channel pulses. If you find you can't pick up the signal, it might be necessary to move your aerial (your hand), fine-tuning it to the correct position. The practitioner's hand might not receive messages from the Primary Channels if the wrist is turned so that the thumb is the highest part of the hand presented. The area of the hand closest to the ceiling should be the thenar eminence. The dorsal aspect of the wrist should be flat to the table; with gravity attracting the artery toward the bone, not the tendons.

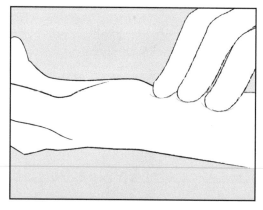

When blockages arise in the Primary Channels they cause the pulses to show either a marked excess or deficiency. If you cannot find a pulse in a given position, the transmission of the signal is jammed. The vibration the organ is sending out to the channel and further to the pulse is not showing up in the pulse because there is a blockage in transmission preventing the externalization of Qi from that organ. If the pulse is missing at the six bean level, there is a blockage of Qi of the Yang organ; on the deep level, at 12 beans of pressure, there is a blockage in the Qi of the Yin organ. Blockages can also cause the pulses to be in a state of excess. This occurs when their Yin-Yang paired organ is blocked and they are trying to compensate.

The compromised flow of Qi manifests as imbalances in organ function even if the organ itself is not impacted, simply because the Qi emanating from the organ is not moving effectively and not able to fully maintain the connections it should be making with other channels and organs.

A blockage must be located and released. It is important to understand that while beneficial, the purpose of this initial treatment is to allow the pulse to show more clearly; this permits the main pulse reading and treatment. Treating the Primary Channels frees the Qi that is flowing to and from the organs and hence frees the signal the Zang Fu is transmitting. Releasing blockages frees the external pathways, creating harmonization between Yin and Yang in the Channels, hence restoring the pulse. It's important to clear these fullnesses or blockages in the chest and then return to the pulse to be able to get a clear view of organ function.

There are several sites in the body where Qi becomes blocked and is prevented from externalizing. The area most commonly indicated is the chest because it is the axis of Qi and Blood; it's where Qi and Blood are mobilized. The *Nan Jing* clinicians would say that the Jing-Well points are where Qi externalizes and comes to the surface. These points can be used to treat fullness felt underneath or in the chest. Indeed this is one of my preferred methods. The theory of the roots and terminations tells us that SP-1 opens up CV-12, LR-1 opens up CV-17 (and CV-18) and KI-1 opens up CV-22 and CV-23. A quick visit to these points can release enough of the blockage to allow entrée to the pulse proper. The pulses should then emerge, especially at the cun position. Anatomically, the cun represents the chest region.

Qi might not be able to come up and out because it is jammed in the floating ribs or the lateral costal area and its resident Mu points. Mu points occur on an energetic continuum that extends from the abdomen and floating ribs up into the chest via the ribcage itself. When constricted, the ribcage can jam transmission between the Zang Fu and the pulses. Tightness in the other Mu points on the torso should be palpated and is confirmed by tightness in the guan position. Tightness in the substernal region at around CV-14 can produce a blockage in the Heart Channel. Tightness in the Liver Mu point, LR-14 can produce blockages in the Liver Channel.

Other key areas of blockage, where the transmission can become jammed include the area beneath the sternum (the solar plexus), the abdomen, lumbar region, throat, limbs and knees. Palpate or ask questions about these areas if you find the pulses to be absent or in a state of excess. Treatment of the Primary Channels can address blockages in any of these anatomical regions.

Sometimes when you're taking the pulse you can feel you're receiving too much information to assimilate. There can be too much "noise" in the pulse, preventing you tuning into it. The pulse can feel as though it wants to jump out of the artery. All this would be considered excess.

Chapter One of scroll two the *Mai Jing* discusses harmonization of these imbalances. The treatments are relatively simple. If there is an excess, the same channel is used to release that excess; if there is a deficiency, the opposite channel (the Yin-Yang paired channel) is used. In very basic terms we are looking for excess pulses: full, tight or wiry pulses, and deficient pulses: very weak, empty or absent pulses. These qualities are determined by examining all the parameters of the pulse—height, width, length, tempo and texture— as they all reflect degrees of excess and deficiency. For example, if you found that the Gallbladder pulse showed excess qualities, if it were, for example, big, rapid and wiry, and bulging out of its position, you would treat the Gallbladder Channel and relieve that excess.

The point most commonly used in this type of treatment was the Shu-Stream point. The Shu-Stream point deals with exterior-interior relationships which are a key function of the Primary Channels. You would also palpate the channel and reduce points that were felt to be tight. After the treatment, when you check the left guan position at six beans of pressure and then press into the Yuan level, you should find a relative sense of balance in the pulses, a sense of evenness throughout the pulse. In this case, the Gallbladder should no longer feel exuberant or full.

(Note: If the Heart is in excess, you would treat the Pericardium Channel, not the Heart Channel directly.)

If, by contrast, there is vacuity in the Gallbladder pulse (guan position at six beans), instead of treating the Gallbladder Channel you would treat the Liver Channel. The Liver Channel would be palpated to locate the points that have the sensation of vacuity, flaccidity or emptiness. Those points would be tonified. Upon checking the pulses after treatment, a sense of balance should be found throughout the levels of the pulse. If not, more palpation should yield more weak points which would then be treated until the change was exacted. Yuan-Source points can also be used in the tonification of the channel.

While treatment of the channels of the left wrist pulse positions generally involve the Shu-Stream points: SI-3, PC-7, GB-41, LR-3, BL-65 and KI-3, often the prescriptions for treatment on the channels of the right wrist pulse positions can be different. These are discussed below. The *Ling Shu* tells us to choose points according to the season, pairing late summer with Ying-Spring points, Spring with Jing-Well points, Autumn with Jing-River points and Winter with He-Sea points. One could choose the Shu-Stream point because the Shu-Stream point is a harmonizer.

EXAMINING THE PRIMARY CHANNEL PULSES

The left wrist reflects the degree to which the body is able to keep a pathogen latent. The right wrist demonstrates the body's capacity to resist a pathogen. In examining the Primary Channels we are registering the way in which pathology is affecting the internal arena. If you were looking for external pathogenic factors affecting the exterior, you would examine the Sinew pulses at three beans of pressure, looking for excesses. The Primary Channels, being channels of the flesh, are deeper, beginning at six beans. We are looking for both excesses and deficiencies at six and twelve beans of pressure.

Treatment involves harmonizing the Yin-Yang pairs. I've included the treatment strategies from the *Mai Jing*. The immediacy of their effectiveness is staggering.

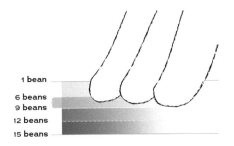

If the pulse is frail, weak or absent at between six and nine beans of pressure, the Yang organ of that position is deficient. If this happens in:

the left cun position, the Small Intestine is deficient. Palpate the navel region to locate pain. This could indicate Shan disorder (accumulations in the Lower Jiao). Palpate and treat the Pericardium Channel (not the Heart Channel) by tonifying its Source point. Also palpate the substernal region and treat sensitivity found there.

the left guan position, the Gallbladder is deficient. There is stagnation at the knees. Ask about knee pain, stiffness or tension of the knee. Release tension and stagnation around the knees, either with local points or with a Sinew treatment. Deficiency in the Gallbladder is known classically to produce a bitter taste in the mouth. According to the *Mai Jing*, LR-2 is indicated for Gallbladder deficiency, rather than LR-3.

the left chi position, the Bladder is deficient. In women you would ask about menstrual irregularities. In men, you would inquire about any type of seminal loss, overindulgence in sex, or dribbling urination, depending on the patient's age. Young children with this pulse may be wetting the bed. Cold limbs are a symptom of both excess and deficiency of the Bladder.

the right cun position, the Large Intestine is deficient. Palpate for substernal tension and for fluid accumulation in the solar plexus, the region inferior to the medial anterior ribcage. This fluid can also manifest as mucus that rattles in the chest. Classically this is sometimes called Water Qi underneath the Heart. This symptom is common to deficiency of the Large Intestine and fullness of the Heart. Coughing is a sign of deficiency of the Large Intestine. Treat LU-9.

the right guan position, the Stomach is deficient. There may be abdominal fullness, heaviness in the abdomen and diarrhea. The point to treat the deficiency is the Luo point, SP-4.

the right chi position, in Primary Channel diagnosis, the Bladder is deficient (as it was in the left chi). The principal sign is cold feet. Regardless of gender, fertility is negatively impacted with this pulse. Triple Heater is unable to fully disseminate Essential Qi and the ability to conceive is compromised.

PRIMARY CHANNEL PULSES REVEALING WEAKNESS IN THE YIN ORGANS

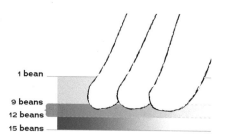

If the pulse is frail, empty and weak at between nine and twelve beans of pressure, the Yin organ of that position is deficient. If this happens in:

the left cun position, the Heart is deficient. There may be chest pain, Heart pain or mouth ulcers. Treat by tonifying flaccid points on the Small Intestine Channel.

the left guan position, the Liver is deficient. Look for pain by palpating the flanks, the lateral costal region, and the area around CV-3. Ask questions about urination difficulty, blockage of urine, nighttime urination or enuresis. Palpate the Gallbladder Channel with a focus on the antique points. Tonify flaccid points.

the left chi position, the Kidneys are deficient. Ask questions pertaining to exhaustion, consumption or taxation of Qi. Ask to see the soles of the feet. They may be very red as a result of the Heat that consumed the Qi, or dry in the aftermath of Heat.
the right cun position, the Lungs are deficient. There can be coughing or dyspnea. There could be stubborn Bi-obstruction in the throat. There could be belching. Find deficient points on the Large Intestine Channel and treat them.

the right guan position, the Spleen is deficient. Look for lower abdominal pain that radiates to the lower back and the lumbar region. The key sign is low back pain originating from the abdomen. Palpate the Stomach channel and find the point of deficiency.

the right chi position, the Kidney and Pericardium are deficient. Symptoms are cold feet and chest pains, respectively. The *Mai Jing* mentions that the patient might be experiencing a lot of dreaming perhaps about the deceased or of water. Palpate the Triple Heater Channel for weak points and treat them. Anatomically, the right chi reflects the area of the Large Intestine and the Kidney region; there may be weakness showing up there, also.

PRIMARY CHANNEL PULSES REVEALING EXCESS IN THE YANG ORGANS

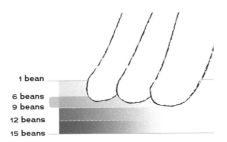

If the pulse has excess qualities (a tight or wiry quality) at between six and nine beans of pressure, the Yang organ of that position has excess Qi. If this is found in:

the left cun position, the Small Intestine has excess Qi. There may be distention in the abdomen. Treat the Shu-Stream point of the Small Intestine.

the left guan position, the Gallbladder has excess Qi. Palpate the abdomen (not the flanks) for abdominal tightness. Release these areas locally and re-examine the pulse. If it is not released, treat the Shu-Stream point, GB-41.

the left chi position, the Bladder is in a state of fullness. Ask questions about the hands or feet getting cold easily and whether there is lateral costal pain. This pain is caused by tight Kidney energetics affecting the Mu point at the base of the ribcage. If the Bladder is deficient, there may still be cold hands and feet.
the right cun position, the Large Intestine is in a state of excess. The patient will likely have pain somewhere. It could be sharp or severe. Examples would be severe pain in the shoulder, intestines or headaches. LI-5 is treated.

the right guan position, the Stomach is in a state of excess. There may be chopstick Qi, also known as the hidden beam, meaning tension in rectus abdominis. Palpate the abdomen, locate the hidden beam and reduce it, needling very superficially. The point to release this excess is the Source point, ST-42.

the right chi position, Dampness has settled in from the Middle Jiao and is putting pressure on the Lower Jiao, creating lower back pain. There is pressure to release Dampness.

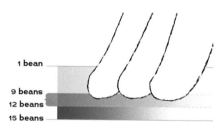

If the pulse has excess qualities (exuberant, full, tight, wiry) at between nine and twelve beans of pressure, the Yin organ of that position has excess Qi. If this happens in:

the left cun position, there is excess Qi in the Heart. Check for fullness beneath the chest (the area of the solar plexus). This presentation is sometimes referred to as "water under the chest", meaning turbidity and Dampness. Palpate to locate the area that feels very Damp. It could feel soggy or swampy. It is likely there is accompanying anxiety. To release the excess, needle PC-7 pointed distally. (Treat the Pericardium rather than the Heart directly.) Or palpate the Pericardium Channel, locate points along the channel that are excess and reduce them.

the left guan position, there is excess Qi in the Liver. Ask about muscular cramping or spasms. Palpate the Liver Channel to locate areas or points of excess and needle to release the musculature, harmonizing the Liver pulse.

the left chi position, there is excess Qi in the Kidneys. There is likely loss of sensory acuity or loss of function in the sensory orifices and the brain. There could be tinnitus or a decline in vision. Memory may be adversely affected. Blood pressure may be elevated. Fullness in the Kidney position can often be found in the elderly. Palpate the Kidney Channel to locate areas of tightness, needle to reduce them and needle KI-3.

the right cun position, the Lungs have excess Qi. The Lungs are unique; they are the only organ that both ascends and descends. The Lungs' ascending function is usually referred to as diffusion, and the descending function is usually referred to in terms of Kidneys grasping Lung Qi. The Lungs must descend the Qi in order for the Kidneys to be able to grasp it, since the Kidneys do not ascend. If the Lungs have exceeded their limit, that is, if they are overrun by pathology, the pulse can be full, floating and long. These pulses can occur in both the superficial and the deep level, since the functions of the Lungs is to ascend and descend. Excess Qi in the Lungs manifests as shortness of breath, dyspnea and chest distention and fullness. There may also be shoulder and chest pain. To release the excess, needle LU-9 pointed distally. Palpate the Lung Channel, locate points along the channel that are excess and reduce them.

the right guan position, there is excess Qi in the Spleen. There may be constipation. Palpate the Stomach channel, focussing on the antique points. Release points that feel as though they have excess Qi. Reduce SP-3.

the right chi position, there is excess Qi in the Pericardium and the Kidneys. There can be lower back pain. This back pain is differentiated from the back pain caused by fullness of the Bladder in that it is felt all the way down to the bone. Bone pain in general can be seen as the fullness of the Kidney Primary Channel. Release KI-3 and/or PC-7.

LUO CHANNEL PULSES

The Luo Channels are implicated if a pathogenic factor has penetrated beyond the Primary Channels and occupies the Blood. According to Chapter 22 of the *Ling Shu*, the Luo Channels are diagnosed by looking and by palpation. Although accurate Luo diagnoses can be attained by looking and palpating alone (indeed, my preferred method) it is possible to gain insight into the body's capacity for latency at the Blood level by examining the pulses.

To determine the required treatment of the Luo Channels from the pulse, we are interested in the interface of Ying and Wei Qi. This is at six beans of pressure. There we can see the capacity of the body to pass Luo pathology up to the Wei level for eradication. If the pulse here is wide, the body likely has enough Ying Qi to hold the pathology in the Luo Channels. If the Luo Channels are active in holding pathology, you will find qualities associated with stagnation (tightness) at six beans of pressure. This is because the Luos are reservoirs of latency with their principal task being to hold pathology and keep it away from the Yuan-Source level and the organs. Along with the stagnation at six beans of pressure, you can find fullness if the Luos are trying to use their mediumship, Blood, to move pathology up to the Wei level for eradication.

Incidentally, measuring from three beans down to six beans tells us how Wei Qi is adjusting to Ying Qi, indicating how well Wei Qi is able to support Ying Qi. Measuring from nine beans up to six beans tell us how Ying Qi is adjusting to Wei Qi, indicating how well Ying Qi can transform into Wei Qi.

If the pulses are floating and empty, there is not sufficient Wei Qi to eliminate a pathogenic factor. The factor has penetrated beyond the level of the Yang Sinews and is either moving into the Yin Sinews or into the Luo Channels. The Yin Sinew Channels and the Luo

Channels are both found at six beans of pressure. Generally, if the Lungs are not diffusing Qi or are floating and empty the pathogen might go to the Yin Sinews first and then perhaps to the Luo Channels. If the pulses are flooding in the right cun position, the pathogen is going to the Luo Channels.

If the pulses are flooding (floating, strong and rapid), the pathogenic factor, combined with the heat the body raised to fight it, is overflowing or spreading and entering the Blood level. The body must create reservoirs to absorb that relative excess. These reservoirs are the Luo points and Luo channels. This process is the transmission of a pathogen from the Wei level into the Ying (Blood) level. As this happens, the face may become ruddy or flushed, the tongue may become very red, the eyes may be bloodshot, the nose bleeding. These are signs of exuberant Heat and Heat in the Blood, which are Luo Channel issues.

If the pulses are rough or choppy, a Blood deficiency is present. This will affect the way a pathogenic factor moves deeper. After the Lungs have failed to expel a pathogen, the Heart steps in to move Blood to expel Wind. A sweat ensues. (This is why sweat is the fluid of the Heart.) If the Blood is insufficient to expel Wind, the pathogenic factor can move into the Blood itself. This is an example of the pathogen manifesting in the cun position (in Tai Yang), but instead of going to Shao Yang it moves into the Blood level because there is not enough Blood to resist it. Luo Channel issues emerge at this point.

If the Lung pulse is not diffusing, the pathogenic factor is free to move to the Yin Sinews and then to the Blood level.

If Wei Qi is lacking integrity resulting in a tight or leathery pulse, the pathogenic factor may move to the Blood level.

If the pulse is tight indicating Cold and pain (slow and tight), or if the pulse is scattered indicating rebellious Qi, the pathogen may go to the Luo Channels as they are channels for the latency of rebellious Qi.

If the pulse is hollow and leathery, Ying Qi is failing to support Wei Qi. The weakness at the Ying level, combined with insufficient Wei Qi, results in the pathogen moving to the Luo Channels.

LUO PULSE REFLEXOLOGY

The Luo Channels are each an extension of their related Primary Channel. Therefore, the pulse positions of the Luo Channels are the same as for the organs. The guan position is of particular interest because it reflects a major part of the Blood arena. However, it gets more detailed than that. If you find a floating, empty and choppy pulse in the guan position, the propensity for a pathogen to go to Shao Yang is high. So too is the likelihood that a pathogen will go to the Gallbladder or Liver Luo. The passage the pathology is taking to the Luo Channels is also easily determined through visual examination of the Luo Channels—finding spider veins along the trajectory.

YIN LUO PULSES AND YANG LUO PULSES

Luo Channels are involved in containing pathology in the Ying level and moving it up to the surface in capillaries for eradication. Hence, Luo pulses are diagnosed at the juncture of the Ying and Wei levels, at six beans of pressure. The action of the finger in Luo diagnoses is a tiny movement upward from nine to six beans of pressure and another action downward from three to six beans of pressure.

If the pulse becomes tight while lifting the finger from nine to six beans of pressure, pathology of the Yin Luo of that position is indicated. For example, if the right cun pulse becomes tight while raising of the finger from nine to six beans of pressure, pathology of the Lung Luo Channel is indicated.

If the pulse becomes tight while pressing down from three to six beans of pressure, pathology of the Yang Luo of that position is indicated. For example, if the right cun pulse becomes tight while pressing the finger from three to six beans of pressure, pathology of the Large intestine Luo Channel is indicated.

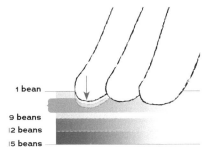

Luo Channels can also be implicated if a bifurcated pulse is present, that is, if two pulses are felt in the same finger position. Differentiate Yin from Yang Luos by applying and noting changes in tightness with pressure as explained above.

Alternative Luo Pulse:

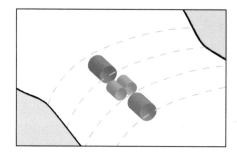

EMPTIED LUO CHANNEL PULSES

Historically, Luo Channels are diagnosed by visibly examining the channels, looking for spider veins. Palpation of the channels is also important, since presence of nodules indicates the Luo Channels have emptied their pathology into the Primary Channel. Often no visible spider veins are found, but nodules of a great variety can be found, ranging from large (perhaps the size of your thumb knuckle), down to the size of a grain of sand. If the pulses are thin and tight or weak and tight at six beans, the Luo Channel is said to have emptied.

TRANSVERSE LUO CHANNEL PULSES

Transverse Luo pathology results in Heat in the organs. Transverse Luos could be said to be indicated if the Yuan level of the pulse is rapid, indicating Heat affecting the organ; Heat has moved from the Luo Channel to the Source level.

DIVERGENT CHANNEL AND EIGHT EXTRAORDINARY PULSES

Divergent Channel and Eight Extraordinary Channel pulses are found at 15 beans of pressure (at the Yuan level) because they deal with issues pertaining to the constitution. The Extraordinary Channels can hold pathology at the constitutional level. The Divergent Channels bring pathology up from the Yuan level to the Wei level for release, or from the Wei level down to the Yuan level for latency.

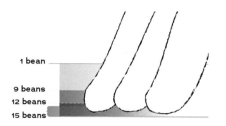

HIDDEN PULSES

Divergent Channel and Eight Extraordinary Channel pulses are fu-hidden pulses. A hidden pulse is one that is revealed after the pulse has been completely pressed down into the bone, stopping all pulsation in the radial artery. This amount of pressure is defined as 15 beans. A hidden pulse indicates there is pathology being held in fu-latency; the pathology itself is being hidden.

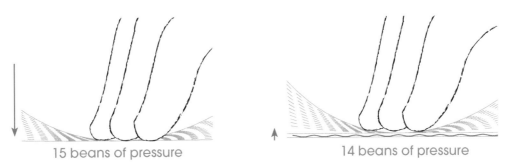

15 beans of pressure   14 beans of pressure

Sometimes it is taught that the bone needs to be stimulated in a more substantial way to yield the hidden pulse. The level of the bone is considered the stone or rock level, and to uproot a rock one must get underneath it and rock it back and forth. Therefore, often the bone is jostled. The fingers press hard and crisscross over the bone, rocking and shaking it in order to get the hidden pulse to emerge. The fingers are then rested at the deep level while the practitioner awaits the emergence of the pulse.

MOVING PULSES

Divergent and Eight Extraordinary pulses are also moving pulses. This refers to the moving Qi of the Kidneys. Therefore, moving pulses—even if they appear in the moderate or superficial levels of the pulse indicating loss of latency—are always Yuan level pulses, either Divergent or Eight Extraordinary. Some refer to the movement as constitutional shaking or rattling, even vibrating. Each of these terms is problematic because they imply a faster or more chaotic movement than is most often found. Finding Divergent or Eight Extraordinary pulses is relatively common, but I have only found a hidden pulse that I would describe as shaking or rattling in patients who are extremely ill, or who have heat in the bone (steaming bone syndrome).

To feel a moving pulse:

If we were arbitrarily to number the pulses so that the odd-numbered beats are found in a given position (lateral to the radial artery) and the even-numbered beats are found slightly more medial (but still lateral to the radial artery), we have found a moving pulse. Moving pulses feel as though they are oscillating from side to side about an axis, all lateral to the radial artery.

119

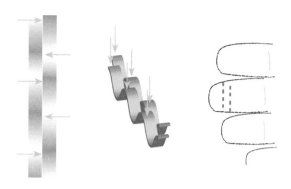

DIVERGENT AND EIGHT EXTRAORDINARY PULSES; DISTINGUISHING BETWEEN THE MOVING PULSES

The Divergent Channels are characterized by hidden pulses because the Divergents are responsible for taking pathology away from the Yuan-Source level to the joints for latency. This is why, once stimulated, the Divergent pulse disappears when it is pressed back to the Yuan-Source level. It shows that the channel is able to draw Qi and move it into the bone level, into the joints. You are interested in the location of these pulses because you want to know whether the patient has the integrity or resources to put the pathogen into latency or to move pathology out of latency. If the Divergent Channel is poised to push the pathogen out of latency, along with a hidden pulse there can be a tight superficial pulse or a superficial floating pulse, indicating the potential for the action of Wei Qi. The channel simply needs releasing using a superficial-deep-superficial treatment.

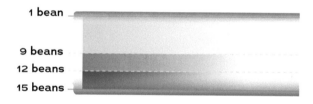

The Eight Extraordinary Channel pulses do not disappear, because the pathology is located in the Yuan level and is not being diverted away from that level. As confirmation, the Eight Extraordinary pulses are not accompanied by a tight pulse in the Wei level.

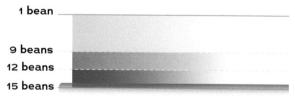

Often, if a Divergent treatment is indicated, there can be at first inquiry very little information showing in the pulse of that position. However, after pressing into the bone and releasing a tiny amount of pressure, a substantial pulse can be revealed.

The method for revealing hidden pulses is as follows:

1. Rest the fingers at between one and three beans of pressure. Note the presence of a tight pulse if there is one.

2. Slowly move all three fingers to pulse neutral position (move cun and guan positions to the moderate level and chi position to the deep level) noting the pulse behaviors on the way.

3. Keep moving the fingers down into the Yuan level. Go to 15 beans of pressure (press enough to occlude the flow of blood in the artery so that all pulsation in the radial artery has ceased and then go a little deeper, as though you are pressing into the bone).

4. Release the tiniest amount of pressure to arrive at 14 beans of pressure. Movement may be felt. (A tiny pulsation that almost feels like a waveform will be felt in the radial artery at 14 beans.)

5. Note where the moving pulses are. When you're first learning, it might feel like pressure against a finger. When you concentrate on it further, you'll feel it is not striking your finger at exactly the same place every time. The sensation could be present at more than one finger.

6. Return all fingers to the bone again by resuming 15 beans of pressure.

7. Findings: Note whether the pulse that appeared after you released pressure from the bone and went up to 14 beans (the hidden pulse) is present as a pulsation in the bone after you press back down to 15 beans.

Once back at 15 beans of pressure:

a. If the moving pulse/s empties (disappears) or dissipates away, a Divergent Channel pulse has been found. The Divergent Channel pair related to that location is either capable of holding pathology latent or is actually holding pathology latent.

b. If the moving pulses remain, an Eight Extraordinary Channel pulse has been found, meaning that the patient is experiencing an Eight Extraordinary Channel disturbance that may benefit from appropriate treatment. Eight Extra pulses can also appear during a major life transition or event; treatment might not be needed.

c. If a pulse appears in the Yuan level only at the second visit to 15 beans, either an Eight Extraordinary Channel or a Divergent Channel has been found. Corroborate signs and symptoms to determine which to treat.

d. If you found a Divergent pulse and during step 1 you found a tight superficial pulse in the Wei level, Wei Qi is active in trying to move the pathogen outward via the Divergent Channel, or the Divergent Channel is losing its capacity to keep the pathogen latent.

DIVERGENT PULSE MAP

The pulse position (cun, guan or chi) at which the hidden pulse disappeared in step 5 above tells you where the patient's latent factors are. It tells you which Divergent Channel is most active in generating latency. A series of superficial-deep-superficial treatments of the confluence indicated would produce a welcome healing crisis as long as the bowels are free. A series of deep-superficial-deep treatments of the confluence indicated would help to ensure that the body can continue to maintain the latency by producing more of the medium related to that confluence.

Since the Divergent Channels are offshoots of the Primary Channels at the Zang Fu, they are found in the pulses according to the Primary Channel map.

RIGHT	LEFT
LI/LU	SI/HT
ST/SP	GB/LR
TH/PC	BL/KI

For example, if you pressed to 15 beans and released to 14 beans and found a moving pulse at the left guan position and then pressed back into 15 beans and experienced the pulse disappearing, you have located a Gallbladder and Liver Divergent Channel issue.

If, in the guan position of either side, the pulse doesn't disappear when you press back to 15 beans, but continues to move around or wriggle, you have found a Dai Mai pulse. (Eight Extraordinary pulses are discussed on page 126.)

A Divergent Channel pulse showing in the left chi position (BL/KI) means that the body has the capacity to hold pathology in the joints and that this process is adequately supported by the Jing.

A Divergent Channel pulse showing in the left guan position (GB/LR) means that the body has the capacity to hold pathology in the joints and that this process is adequately supported by the Blood.

A Divergent Channel pulse showing in the right guan position (ST/SP) means that the body has the capacity to hold pathology in the joints and that this process is adequately supported by the Jin-Thin Fluids.

A Divergent Channel pulse showing in the left cun position (SI/HT) means that the body has the capacity to hold pathology in the joints and that this process is adequately supported by the Ye-Thick Fluids.

A Divergent Channel pulse showing in the right chi position (TH/PC) would indicate loss of capacity to hold latency. Re-establish latency via TH/PC Divergent Channel.

A Divergent Channel pulse finding in the right cun position (LI/LU) would indicate loss of capacity to hold latency (as with the right chi position). Turn attention to establishing latency via TH/PC or LI/LU with some degree of urgency.

SIMPLE DIVERGENT PULSES

If you find a quality in the Wei level that seems to be matched in the Yuan level, it could be said that the Divergent is active in trying to release its pathology. This idea can be validated by testing for hidden pulses.

Historically, the early descriptions of hidden pulses referred to finding a quality at the deep level that is normally expected at the surface. In other words, Yang qualities are found at the Yin levels. The presence of something hiding in its counterpart is the earliest description of a hidden pulse (fu mai/latent pulse). For example, on the Yuan level you might find something that is Yang (big or long). This is a sign of pathology that should be expressed and cleared through the Wei level, but has retreated to the interior. It is another example of latency being evident. As pulse taking became more sophisticated, the technique of pressing into the bone developed. This is the most effective way of diagnosing the Divergent Channels.

It is not compulsory to use Divergent pulses to qualify the use of the Divergent Channels. For example, pathology of the Ye-Thick Fluids occurs at the Heart and Small Intestine Divergent Channel confluence. If you examined the pulses and found issues with Ye-Thick Fluids, you could certainly responsibly use the Heart and Small Intestine Divergent Channels.

INTERNALIZING OR EXTERNALIZING: DEEP-SUPERFICIAL-DEEP OR SUPERFICIAL-DEEP-SUPERFICIAL

Superficial-Deep-Superficial or Deep-Superficial-Deep

The Divergent Channels are shown to be active or potentially active with the disappearance of the pulse at the second visit to 15 beans of pressure. To be active means they are holding pathology latent. To be potentially active means they are capable of making pathology latent.

One way to determine whether a Divergent Channel is internalizing pathology (making pathology latent) or externalizing pathology (moving pathology out of latency) is to check

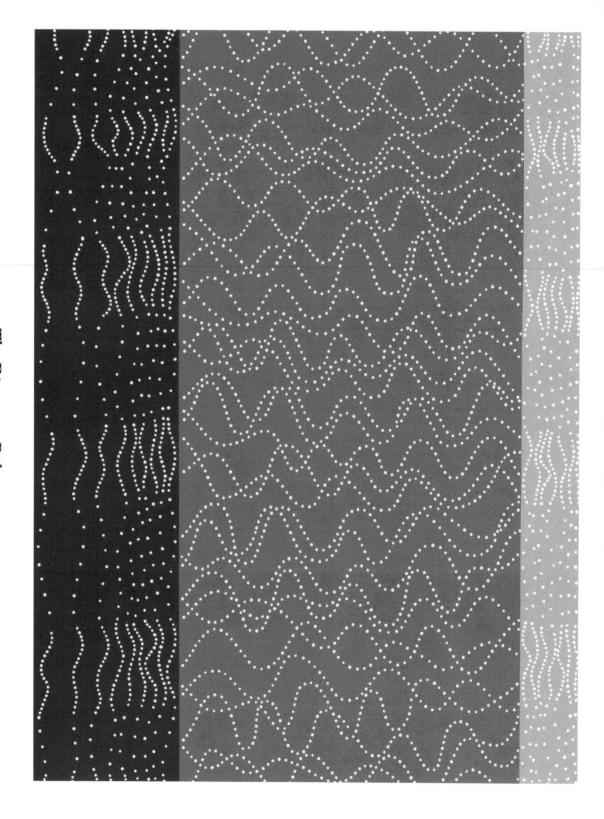

The Divergent Pulse

The Divergent Channels are present to preserve humanity. When a particular tightness in the Wei level is reflected in the Yuan level, the body may be trying to bring a pathogen into latency, or to shift one out of latency. Here we see in the Ying level that life is continuing in a joyful way with organs unencumbered, while the body works behind the scenes, deftly hiding the pathogen that would otherwise threaten the body's equilibrium.

to see whether there is a floating Triple Heater pulse. See Appendix I, page 195. If there is a floating Triple Heater pulse, the Divergent Channel diagnosed (it could be in any pulse position) is failing to hold onto latency. If something is coming out of latency, the Divergent pulse found can be very strong at 14 beans.

The same channel could possibly be used to hold onto pathology, but would need help doing so. A deep divergent treatment would be performed.

FREQUENTLY ASKED QUESTIONS

1. My patient has several Divergent Channel pulses. Is this normal?

Divergent pulses show the location of the body's capacity for latency, so you may find them mostly at the level of the left chi and both guan positions because the first three confluences, the BL/KI, GB/LR and ST/SP are the most prominent areas of latency. GB/LR divergent pulses indicate that the body is using blood to maintain the latency, but a blood deficient or anemic person, for example, doesn't have the resources of blood to maintain latency and so that person will not have a GB/LR Divergent pulse. They might hold on to pathology through ST/SP instead. Divergent pulses are not constitutional in the sense of always being there. If you do not have enough fluid, you are not going to have a ST/SP Divergent pulse. The more divergent pulses you can find, the better the body's capacity of holding on to latency because it has various resources with which to hold on. If you can only find one, that means that the body is already under a lot of taxation. Divergent pulses manifesting indicate the availability of resources at that time.

2. I found Divergent and Eight Extraordinary pulses on the same wrist. Is that possible?

Yes. If, for example you found moving pulses at both the guan and chi positions and when you pushed them back to 15 beans the guan disappeared and the chi continued to be even stronger, you have found that Gallbladder and Liver Divergent Channels are capable of holding latency and that there is concurrently a Yin Qiao Mai pulse.

3. When I was pressing back to 15 beans, I found a Stomach and Spleen divergent pulse but at the same time, a pulse appeared at the chi position. How do I know whether this is a Yin Qiao Mai pulse or a Triple Heater Pericardium pulse?

To decide, corroborate those findings with the signs and symptoms. Incidentally, often on the left wrist the pulse on deeper investigation shows a Bladder and Kidney Divergent pulse. This is because the body, if capable, may ultimately attempt to clear the pathology through the first confluence, the Bladder (and Kidney) Divergent Channels.

EIGHT EXTRAORDINARY CHANNEL PULSES

HISTORICAL REFERENCES TO THE EIGHT EXTRAORDINARY CHANNEL PULSES

Wang Shu He's Pulse Classic and the *Nan Jing* both explain that the 27 channels (15 of the 16 Luo Channels plus the 12 channels we often call Primary) cannot reach the Eight Extraordinary Channels because these special channels have their own independent level. Chapter 27 of the *Nan Jing* says, "The ancient sages [the Kidneys] constructed ditches and reservoirs for the waterways [the Primary Channels] in the event of something extraordinary [the overflow of resources or overflow of pathology]. When rain pours down from Heaven [events beyond our control], the ditches and reservoirs [the Eight Extraordinary Channels] become full. The ditches are beyond reach of the Primary Channels." This means that surplus resources are stored in the Eight Extras but the 12 Primary Channels can't access that richness (in good health) or the pathology (in compromised health). Hence, the pulses of the Eight Extraordinary Channels are felt at a level beyond those of the other channels. Because they carry constitutional Qi, they are felt only at the deep level of the pulses.

The theory of the Eight Extraordinary pulses was systematized in the Ming Dynasty by Li Shi Zhen, one of the greatest compilers of information in Chinese medical history and owner of a large library of medical texts. Much earlier, in the Han Dynasty, Wang Shu He's description of the Eight Extra pulses was limited because at the time he wrote, the Eight Extra Channels were not used in clinical treatments. A fundamental shift occurred during the Song Dynasty as the influential philosopher Zhu Xi wrote that Ming-Destiny is malleable, not entirely fixed by heaven. Physicians saw in this a shift, a change in the way the Eight Extra Channels could be used. As they sought to implement this new view, they began to tap into destiny and its carrier, Jing. At this point, the Eight Extras ceased being viewed only as channels of transformation and began to be seen as channels of intervention.

THE SENSATION OF THE EIGHT EXTRAORDINARY PULSES

Because the Eight Extra Channels are ditches (sites where the body can hold pathology latent) they have Fu-Hidden Pulses. Li Shi Zhen refers to these pulses as having a vibrating quality about them. The word moving is perhaps more apt because word vibrate implies buzzing, as in the vibration of an electric shaver or a bee. This is not what is meant by vibrating. In the context of the Eight Extra pulses, the words moving and vibrating are intended to mean the same thing, that is, the pulse wants to move away from your finger. It doesn't want to stay under your finger. The pulses feel a little uncomfortable being where they are and so they move, usually laterally with alternating beats close to and away from the tendon. As you first encounter the pulse, the first beat might begin on one side of the finger, say lateral to the finger, but with the next beat the pulse is felt to the other side of the finger to the medial side. It will continue to oscillate back and forth between either side of the finger as though it is unable to stay under your finger and is trying to move away from it by moving toward and away from the tendon. As they are hidden pulses, they are felt after pressure has been applied to the bone (explained later).

The presence of Eight Extra pulses does not necessarily indicate pathology. The nature of these pulses may merely be reflecting the moving Qi of the Kidneys, or the availability or depth of Yuan Qi.

In my practice I often find that if an Eight Extra Channel is indicated, the postnatal pulses (the pulses at the Ying and Wei levels) become less prominent and the pulses at the Yuan level start to move, even before I have palpated the bone to prepare to look for hidden pulses. I used to think this happened because I love the Eight Extra channels, but increasingly I see that patients will present the information we need in order for them to receive the treatment most suited to them. Eight Extra Channel pulses can emerge when I'm half expecting to find something completely different. To be a blank slate as a practitioner, to suspend expectation, to have unbiased investigation, is very important. To hear the patient's pulses as though you've never taken that person's pulses before is to be truly listening. If, as you are taking the pulses, you notice that they start to sway from side to side under your fingers, look at the Eight Extra pulses in the bone level even if you weren't planning to. It's likely that you will find a clear and unequivocal diagnosis there.

PRACTITIONER INTENTION IN EIGHT EXTRAORDINARY PULSE DIAGNOSIS

While the Wei and Ying level pulses are easily changed through suggestion or the intention of the practitioner, Yuan level pulse changes come only through the patient's own cultivation or intention. This is because the Yuan level contains the destiny. Though partly divinely predetermined and partly determined by the individual, the Yuan level is not in the practitioner's actionable domain. The practitioner can, however, without breech of ethics, intend to clarify the patient's perception of his or her own destiny simply by holding a space of endless possibilities as they take the pulse.

STIMULATING THE EIGHT EXTRAORDINARY PULSES: ROCKING THE PULSE

Although the Eight Extraordinary pulses are at the Yuan level, there are gradations of accessibility for the practitioner. In some patients the Yuan level pulses are readily felt; in others they need to be stimulated. The following steps stimulate the Eight Extraordinary pulse so that it is easier to find. This will prepare the pulses for diagnosis described in the method below. It is not compulsory.

1. Inform your patient that you are pressing deeply into the wrist because you want to gain

access to something deep-seated.

2. Position your three fingers. Press down to nine beans of pressure, the center of the Ying level.

3. Move your fingers lengthwise along the artery a little. Roll them a little as you go. This allows you to feel the position of the radial artery. Some are more medial than others. Note any distortions of the pathway of the artery and adjust your fingers to match. Now roll your fingers across the artery. Feel for its borders. Note whether it is wiry or tight, etc.

4. Slowly press down all the way through the rest of the Ying level and then through the Yuan level. Near the bottom you will occlude the flow of blood through the radial artery. Keep pressing down until you feel you're actually pressing into the bone. This is defined as 15 beans of pressure. This pressure is very substantial.

5. While pressing deeply at the 15 bean level, rock your three fingers back and forth over the bone. This shakes the bone up, encouraging it to reveal the hidden pulses.

6. Release to 14 beans of pressure. Fourteen beans is defined as lifting the tiniest amount of pressure to allow the tiniest vibration to become re-established in the radial artery. A small amount of blood might flow.

7. Look for moving pulses, pulses that are oscillating from side to side. If you find no moving pulses, repeat step 3 once more.

8. If no moving pulses are felt, it doesn't necessarily mean that there are no Eight Extraordinary issues. We all have those. It can, however, mean that the patient is not ready to be treated at the Eight Extraordinary level. To treat at the Eight Extraordinary level when it is neither time to do so nor invited to is considered in acupuncture to be the ultimate form of disrespect to the patient, and is classically considered malpractice.

EIGHT EXTRAORDINARY PULSE TAKING METHOD

1. Ensure the patient's wrist is Positioned flat on something comfortable, not a hard surface.

2. Rest the fingers at the pulse positions.

3. Move all three fingers down slowly into the Yuan level. Go to 15 beans of pressure; press enough to occlude the flow of blood in the artery and then go a little deeper, as though you're pressing right into the bone. This is very significant pressure that will temporarily leave the indentations of your fingers in the flesh at the wrist after you remove them. Note: it shouldn't be so much pressure that it causes pain in the patient.

4. Release the tiniest amount of pressure to arrive at 14 beans of pressure. You'll feel slight movements emerging.

5. Note which pulse is moving or pushing back against a finger. It could be at more than one finger.

6. Press all three fingers into the bone again, returning to 15 beans of pressure.

7. Note whether the pulse or pulses that appeared in step 5 after you released pressure

from the bone (the hidden pulses) are present as a pulsation in the bone at this current revisiting of 15 beans. This pulsation usually manifests as an oscillating, moving pulse in the bone. The pulse, if present, will move laterally and medially about the center of the finger. If the moving pulse is present, you have found an Eight Extraordinary pulse.

8. Roll your fingers distally a little to see whether the cun pulse extends outward and proximally to see whether the chi pulse extends beyond its position.

9. Determine which Eight Extraordinary pulse is present according to the criteria in the section that follows.

10. If you couldn't locate any Eight Extraordinary pulses, stimulate the Eight Extraordinary pulses as described above, on page 127.

EIGHT EXTRAORDINARY PULSE DIAGNOSIS

Note: The order in which these pulses are discussed is simply the order in which I find it easiest to teach them. The order does not echo Eight Extraordinary theory.

Perform all the steps of the Method, above.

If the moving pulse is felt at the:

Cun position only, Yang Qiao Mai is indicated.

Guan position only, Dai Mai is indicated.

Chi position only, Yin Qiao Mai is indicated.

If the pulse is moving and long at the cun position, extending distally toward the thumb, Yang Wei Mai is indicated.

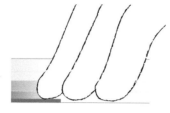

If there are moving pulses in both the cun and guan positions, Yang Wei Mai is indicated.

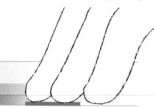

If the pulse moving and long at the chi position, extending proximally toward the elbow, Yin Wei Mai is indicated.

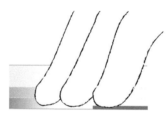

If there are moving pulses in both the guan and chi positions, Yin Wei Mai is indicated.

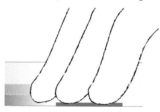

If the pulse is moving in all three positions, you have found a long Eight Extraordinary pulse. There are three possible broad diagnoses here: Ren Mai, Chong Mai and Du Mai. To determine which is showing in the pulse, allow your fingers to release as slowly as possible, together upward toward the surface. You are interested in the point at which you lose the sensation of the long pulse occupying all three positions.

If the moving pulses in all three positions float, following you all the way to within the Wei level, Du Mai is indicated. Du Mai is the Sea of Yang and its hidden pulse will rise up to the most Yang level.

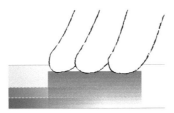

If the moving pulses in all three positions float, following you all the way to within the Ying level but not higher, Chong Mai is indicated. The Chong is the Sea of Blood and mediates between the Yang and the Yin. As a result, the Chong rests at the moderate level.

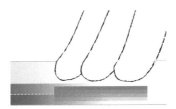

If the moving pulses in all three positions float but you lose contact with all three pulses while still within the Yuan level, Ren Mai is indicated. Ren Mai is the Sea of Yin and is dense and heavy.

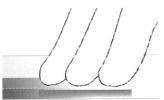

SUMMARY OF EIGHT EXTRAORDINARY PULSE POSITIONS

Perform all the steps of the Method.

If the moving pulse is felt at the cun position only, Yang Qiao Mai is indicated.

If the moving pulse is felt at the guan position only, Dai Mai is indicated.

If the moving pulse is felt at the chi position only, Yin Qiao Mai is indicated.

If the pulse is moving and long at the cun position, extending distally, toward the thumb, or if it is found in both cun and guan positions Yang Wei Mai is indicated.

131

If the pulse is moving and long at the chi position, extending proximally toward the elbow, or it is found in both the guan and chi positions, Yin Wei Mai is indicated.

If the pulses are moving in all three positions and float, following you all the way to within the Wei level, Du Mai is indicated.

If the pulses are moving in all three positions and float, following you all the way to within the Ying level but not higher, Chong Mai is indicated.

If the pulses are moving in all three positions and float but you lose contact with all three pulses while still within the Yuan level, Ren Mai is indicated.

PULSES OF THE ANCESTRIES

In Classical Medicine, the Eight Extraordinary Channels are arranged in three groups called ancestries. The ancestries are arranged in the order in which they allow development to unfold.

The pulses of the first ancestry—the foundational ancestry comprising Chong Mai, Ren Mai and Du Mai—are less often found because they give birth to the other Eight Extraordinary channels. Pathology of the other five channels is generally much more common in the pulses. If Chong, Ren or Du pulses are found, they should be selected for treatment above other findings since the pathology being diagnosed is deeper.

The second ancestry comprises the Wei Channels.

The most commonly found Eight Extraordinary pulses are those of the third ancestry: Yin Qiao Mai, Yang Qiao Mai and Dai Mai. This is because the Qiao's are the repositories of the Luo channels, the containment of all emotional pathology. The Luo Channels connect to the Source and ultimately deposit their pathology in the Qiao's. Dai Mai is a key repository of constitutional waste.

THE CHONG MAI PULSE IN MORE DETAIL

Chong Mai, the Sea of Prenatal Qi is responsible for deriving Yin and Yang, converting Yin and Yang into Blood and Qi and bringing Blood and Qi from the Lower Jiao to the Middle Jiao. After determining that there is a Chong Mai pulse present in the first place, the first and second trajectories can be found to be reflected in the pulse, though subtly. The first trajectory of Chong Mai emerges at the chi and guan positions; the second trajectory is reflected at the cun position. This reflects the anatomical location of the trajectories of the channel; the first trajectory ends at KI-21 and the second extends from there to the Upper Jiao. Issues in specific trajectories will show as a tight or wiry quality in the corresponding positions: the cun reflects the Upper Jiao, the guan the Middle Jiao, and the chi the Lower Jiao.

Chong Mai's dissemination of Yin through Ren Mai and Yang through Du Mai requires freedom in the chest region. Any blockage in this dissemination is considered a disruption of Kidney Qi supporting Spleen Qi. These blockages show in the pulses as a slipperiness when the finger is rolled to palpate between pulse positions (cun and guan or guan and chi) at a deep level. A slipperiness that shows itself when rolling at the deep level between the guan and the cun position likely indicates a blockage in the diaphragm. A slipperiness that shows when rolling at the deep level between the guan and the chi position likely indicates a blockage in Dai Mai. A pulse that is wiry when rolling from the chi to the guan position on a deep level also indicates a disruption. If the guan pulse is also full, you may find that the patient has pain around the navel.

The Chong pulse can also show exuberance in speed or strength, or a scattering quality. The exuberance has a chaotic quality, preventing you from gathering information about the pulse. This means Yang is exuberant and Yin is being expended too quickly. The Jing is being released into a gaseous state, appearing scattered. This shows that there is not enough Yin to anchor or control the momentum of the Chong Mai. This often results in Running Piglet Qi.

When Yang is escaping and there is a Yin deficiency, the Chong may attempt to re-acquire essence since it is responsible for dissemination of Yin and Yang. The reacquisition is reflected on the moderate level. If the moving pulse at the moderate level is thin, tight and slow in all three positions, Chong is trying to conserve Yin. In this case you might find Chong and an accompanying Ren pulse. (You'll find Chong on one wrist, and Ren on the other.)

The transformation of prenatal Qi to postnatal Qi in the Chong is felt as its moderate level pulses are felt to gather (become tight).

CHONG MAI AND THE LEFT AND RIGHT SIDES

Unlike the Ren and the Du, the Chong is a prenatal channel extending into the postnatal arena. If you find the Chong pulse on the right side, you are looking at the Yin aspect of the Chong, that is, Chong as the Sea of Blood. You would focus on using Chong to support Blood.

If you find a Chong pulse on the left side, which is Yang, you are looking at Chong as the Sea of the 12 Primary Channels and the sea of the Zang Fu. In this case, Chong is supporting Qi. A Chong pulse found on the left side calls for moxibustion to tonify Qi.

THE REN MAI PULSE

A Ren pulse may show if there are Yin accumulations with an underlying Yin deficiency or an exuberance of Yang with a relative deficiency of Yin. In presenting a Ren pulse, the body is requesting urgent nourishment of Yin. The deep level is the level of mutual consumption. Here we are seeing that the Yin of the Ren is constantly being burned as fuel to create Yang Qi. If there is insufficient Yin, the Chong can move Yang Qi up too fast, causing Running Piglet Qi. (A Du Mai pulse can sometimes accompany a Ren pulse, but the Ren pulse will show if the body is looking expressly for Yin nourishment in itself, rather than the assistance from Yin for the containment of exuberant Yang.)

All three positions of Ren might be thin, as Yin is depleted. If the Ren issues advance, the pulse might also become tight as the body tries to conserve resources.

Above the Eight Extra pulse arena, in the Ying level in particular, the pulses might concurrently be slippery as the body tries to gather Yin systemically. This can lead to pathological accumulations of Yin, leading in turn to the manifesting of the classical symptoms of Ren which include any accumulations in the Lower Jiao. These conditions are collectively referred to as Shan disorders (including hernia, testicular swelling and prostate problems) and Zheng Jia (including fibroids, cysts, endometriosis and mobile or immobile masses).

If the moderate level is weak and tight, there may be a severe Qi deficiency. The Ren might be trying to support Yang Qi. If this is the case, the tongue may not be red and yet the pulses will be rapid. This is because the Kidney Yang is unable to support the Spleen; Chong is stepping in to convert the Yin of Ren into Yang to provide for the Spleen.

Later, as more mediumship is lost, Yin Wei Mai attempts to gather back Yin and Blood, and Yang Wei Mai attempts to gather back Yang to relieve the pressure on the Chong to move out more Yin and Yang.

THE DU MAI PULSE

Being the Sea of Yang, the Du Mai Pulse can have extremes of all of the pulse parameters. Height, width, length, tempo and texture can all be in relative excess. Du Mai sits very high in the pulse. It can be wide, it is very long, extending through all three positions, and it can be tight or wiry. The pulse is uncomfortable being under your finger and wants to move. Stiffness along the spine is a classical symptom of Du Mai and should be addressed.

If the pulse scatters as it floats, Yang is being lost. Yang must not surge too quickly. If the Du pulse is tight and rapid, Yang is exuberant. It is being expressed too quickly and it is likely that Wind is present. There might therefore be seizures and convulsions, or in children, Fright-Wind.

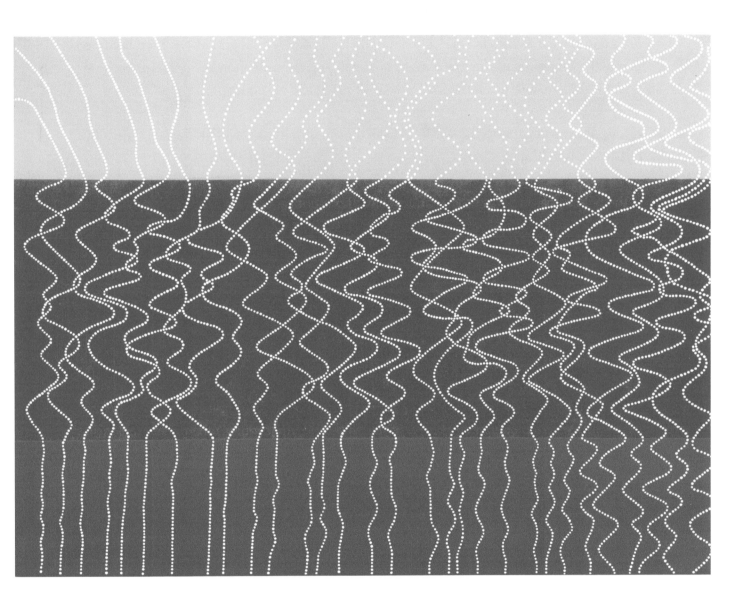

The Ecstatic Pulse

This work shows the three distinct divisions felt in the pulses at the wrist during the practice of diagnosis. The bottom region relays to the practitioner the readiness of the Heart to accept and carry out the Divinely bestowed blueprint of one's life. The blueprint, encrypted in the constitutional level at conception and cemented at birth, ripples through the bones, imprinting itself in the Blood—the mediumship of physical existence—via its connection with the bone marrow. Here we see that with the passage of time the blueprint is embraced, enacted enthusiastically in the Blood, then informs the top region—that of personal space and unspoken interaction—with the notion that to follow one's Divine plan creates a joy that is universal

REN SECOND TRAJECTORY AND DU SECOND TRAJECTORY: LEFT AND RIGHT SIDE DIFFERENTIATION

Ren and Du are stores of prenatal Yin and Yang, respectively. Prenatally, the right Kidney is Yang and the left Kidney is Yin. Very often the Du Mai pulse is found on the right because prenatally Yang manifests on the right. The Ren Mai pulses will often be on the left because prenatally Yin manifests on the left. This is all regardless of gender.

Therefore:

If the pulses are floating to the Wei level in all three positions on the right, the first trajectory of Du Mai is indicated.

If the pulses float to within the Yuan level in all positions on the left, the first trajectory of Ren Mai is indicated.

However, Du Mai has a trajectory (the second) that generates the Ren Channel. If the pulses are floating to the Wei-defensive level in all three positions on the left, the second trajectory of Du Mai is indicated. That pulse is also likely to be big and rapid in all three positions. Yang is being shown to be focusing on the creation of Yin at a constitutional level. The Yang Qi is moving from the first trajectory into the second trajectory to create Yin. Du Mai is trying to support Ren Mai. You would treat the Du Channel using points that engender Yin and Ying, promoting the production of fluids. This is why Du has points to nourish Yin. You could also choose points on the Ren that tonify Yang to help replenish Yang if the Du has been depleted in the process of supporting Ren Mai.

Ren Mai has a trajectory (the second) that generates Du Mai. If a long, deep, moving three-position pulse is found to float within the Yuan level in all positions on the right, the second trajectory of Ren Mai is indicated. Ren is trying to support Du Mai. Yin is transforming into Yang, trying to help Du Mai generate Yang Qi. Yin Qi is moving from the first trajectory into the second trajectory to create Yang. If you find a Ren Mai pulse on the right side, you are still treating the Ren channel but you are treating the Ren Channel's capacity to give birth to the Du channel, using points on the Ren that tonify Yang. This is why Ren has points to tonify Yang. Treat Ren using moxibustion. You could also treat points on the Du that nourish Yin to help replenish Yin if the Ren is depleted in the process of supporting Du Mai.

REN OR DU MAI PULSES WITH AN ACCOMPANYING CHONG MAI PULSE

If the pulses are very strong on the superficial level, and very strong on the deep level, Chong Mai and Du Mai are indicated. There is excess Yang in Du Mai but the origin of Du Mai is Chong. Wang Shu He considers this pulse to show a decline in the mind. This pulse is commonly found in the very elderly; their pulses are very strong on the superficial level and surprisingly, also very strong on the deep level. The constant and normal interplay of transformation where Yang is becoming Yin and Yin is becoming Yang is out of balance and the scales are tipped toward Yin becoming Yang. If this is occurring, the Blood can become depleted, and memories (which are stored in the Blood) are lost to Yang resulting in what is known classically as feeble-mindedness or weakness of memory. The memory (or mind) is breaking up, causing there to be more than one mind. Alzheimer's, dementia, even schizophrenia can result. Consider treating with Chong.

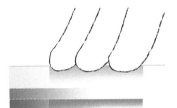

Another Chong and Du combination scenario is when there is an exuberant quality at the deep level extending from the chi to guan positions and also floating exuberant pulses on all the levels. Again, Yuan Qi is moving the Jing too quickly. Personality disorders arise in these cases.

When Chong and Ren are out of balance and presenting at the same time (one on each wrist), Yin is transforming and being lost too quickly. This patient may be very impulsive and unable to gather his or her thoughts.

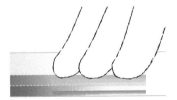

WEI MAI PULSES

The Wei pulses are long pulses. This is reflective of the Wei quality, Wei meaning net or linking (not to be confused with Wei-defensive Qi). The Wei's reach out to collect and restock resources. There is a communication between pulse positions as the Wei Channels throw out their silken net to gather and preserve resources, causing a lengthening of the pulses even to the point of being connected.

In Yang Wei Mai, the gathering function results in pulses that stretch distally as the channel gathers up Yang from the superior anatomy. Yang Wei Mai pulses can be felt to emerge from the guan position and extend upward to the cun and even beyond it into the thenar eminence, or it can emerge at the cun position and extend back toward the guan position. It can be found at the moderate level or be superficial or float.

In Yin Wei Mai the gathering function results in pulses that extend proximally away from the chi position. The Yin Wei Mai pulse extends from the chi toward the elbow, or from the chi toward the guan position, or from the guan toward the chi position. All these pulses have a long, slightly stretched out quality.

Yang Wei Mai is trying to consolidate Yang, using Wei-defensive Qi to support deep Yang Qi. Yin Wei Mai is trying to consolidate Yin to support deep Yin. This is all happening to take pressure off the Chong so that it doesn't have to mete out more prenatal Qi (Yin and Yang). The body is always seeking to preserve these precious resources—for longevity, to maximize the chance of procreation, and to conserve resources to ensure the capacity for latency.

In order to gather resources, as Yang Wei Mai brings Qi back to itself to replenish Yang, and Yin Wei Mai brings Blood back to itself to replenish Yin, the Wei Channels stagnate the Qi and Yin, including Blood. Symptoms therefore also include severe headaches and visual dizziness as Yang Wei collects Yang, leading to a pulse that is full, exuberant and moving to the cun position as it stagnates Yang to gather it. Yang Wei Mai can even flood as the stagnation becomes overwhelming. Symptoms then become those of Qi escaping. In Yang Wei Mai these include dizziness and visual blur. In Yin Wei Mai, this flooding can manifest as hemorrhaging, bleeding, loss of Fluids and Jing. Yin Wei Mai may especially stagnate Blood in the chest, affecting the circulation of Blood in the Heart, causing Heart pain. The Yin Wei pulse reflects this stagnation of Yin so that it feels big, wide and deep in the chi position. It will not float. Yang Wei Mai can float, especially in the heart position, demonstrating the accumulation of Yang. As the gathering action of the Wei's becomes chronic, its moving quality is accentuated.

Note: Wang Shu He believed that if there is a surplus of prenatal qi the body creates "ditches" to absorb the surplus via the Wei Mai. In our culture we tend not to preserve enough prenatal Qi to be able to enjoy this function.

THE EMERGENCE OF QIAO PATHOLOGY FOLLOWING PATHOLOGY OF THE WEI CHANNELS

Periodically there are pauses in life that seem like obstacles but which in fact herald the coming of a major development. The change in question could be graduation, marriage, divorce, career changes, becoming a parent, losing a parent, emigrating, retirement, etc. The mind must join the body in concert to fully assimilate the change. Additionally, there are the natural phases such as puberty, fertility and menopause or andropause. In these natural changes, the body signals to the mind that it should also be changing. Essential to these transformational periods is a time of introspection, of reflection. Pausing is required. If one can't get past these obstacles and embrace change, if the change is not assimilated in the bodymind, the Qiao Channels are affected. Since the Qiao's affect the structure, movement through life is adversely affected if there is resistance to change. The Qiao's cannot present with their characteristic pathology of excess (stagnation) unless there is deficiency set up in the Wei's caused by the failure to stop, reflect and develop.

QIAO MAI AND DAI MAI PULSES

The Eight Extraordinary Channels are able to take overflowing pathogenic factors affecting the constitution and hold them in latency. They are also able to store an overflow of resources (Yin), but this doesn't really happen in our culture because we do not rest, cultivate and enjoy the quietude that is necessary to preserve these resources. If the ditches were not present (and we lived a lifestyle maximizing Yin resources), the body would try to have closure and form resistance to the excess. Wiry pulses would be the norm. This can also happen when the ditches are full.

The channels that deal with surplus Yin and Yang pathologically are the Yin Qiao Mai, Yang Qiao Mai and Dai Mai. In the pulses of these three channels we feel the overflowing of accumulated waste resulting from a long period of pathology and its accompanying stagnation. The channel wants to absorb the pathology back in and drain it but the waste has backed up and begun to emerge; part of the pathology is protruding. You can feel this protrusion in the pulse. In the Qiao pulses and the Dai pulse you feel the pressure of something trying to siphon inward, like putting your hand under a vacuum cleaner nozzle while you resist its suction. It can be very subtle but it's there. This sensation can be found for the excess of Yin (Yin Qiao Mai), the excess of Yang (Yang Qiao Mai), and the Yin and Yang excess combination (Damp-Heat) that is associated with Dai Mai. These channels cannot present healthy pulses.

The Qiao Mai exhibit moving and shaking pulses. They can be engorged or swollen to the point of feeling explosive, as though they want to break loose. In very advanced pathology, they can scatter. Both Qiao's have pulses of excess. This is because the Qiao's reflect the tension that arises in the body as the mind strives for perfection. Perfection is only attainable as a state of mind. The imperfections of daily life must be let go from the mind, but the mind is often not willing to do so. The Qiao's deal with the inconsistencies between the yearning of the mind and life itself, creating tensions in order to create a buffer. That which causes us to feel uncomfortable within ourselves or out in the world is what we dwell on consistently. The *Nan Jing* considers the Qiao's to be giant Luo Channels that deal with the way in which we feel uncomfortable about life. Li Shi Zhen considered the Qiao Mai's to be our parasites, gnawing away at us, causing us to feel contaminated. We don't need to have this contamination because it is the product of our own mind. Hence the Qiao pulses show all this pathology of the bodymind as a full restlessness with an underlying tension.

The Qiao pulses feel like full pulses but are in fact revealing a response to deficiencies set up in the Wei channels.

The *Nan Jing* tells us that the Luo's empty into the Qiao's. The emotional debris set up in the Wei Channels caused by the failure to be reflective, cultivate stillness, connect oneself to one's gut instincts and live accordingly, creates emotional disturbance which overloads the Luo Channels which in turn empty into the Qiao's. The difference is that the Luo vessels are confined to blood vessels and are often very fine while the Qiao's affect one's stance and physical structure. At the structural level, the Qiao's hold a reflection of the emotional stresses caused by the resistance to living one's life purpose. Hence, they produce pulses of excess in response to an underlying weakness. This excess is coming from the draining of the Luo Channels.

The Qiao's are a tandem pair. Hence, if Yang Qiao Mai is in excess (tight or even floating and tight), it follows that Yin Qiao Mai is weak. If Yin Qiao Mai is in excess, it follows that Yang Qiao Mai is weak. If both Qiao pulses show up, one may appear full and tight and the other may be weak, thin or empty. The Qiao's are constantly trying to produce balance, which is why they affect the gait.

Qiao pulses are often shorter pulses as they focus on holding Qi either in the lateral aspect or the medial aspect of the structure. The Yang Qiao Mai is a short, gathering pulse that feels like an excess pulse because it is gathering resources in response to a long-standing deficiency. Yang Qiao Mai tries to provide energy to fill up that short quality but as energy moves out in order to gather it brings the moving Qi of the Kidneys with it. In other words, Triple Heater is affected. At the deep level of the pulse you can feel something moving out. That moving and vibrating quality increases as the channel moves Yang up to the cun position. This is why the principal signs of Yang Qiao Mai are seizures and head Wind. Yin Qiao Mai, in turn, is supporting Yin which has become deficient and short. The Yin Qiao Mai pulse doesn't fill its position (the chi) but it is clearly moving and trying to fill with Yin. This is why the principal sign of Yin Qiao Mai is somnolence.

THE DAI MAI PULSE

Dai Mai integrates Chong, Ren and Du. It keeps the three channels contained and interacting. Dai consolidates, reintegrates and absorbs excess from the Middle Jiao. Therefore its pulse is focused in the guan position.

Just as it is important not to infringe with any Eight Extraordinary Channel, it is very important not to infringe by using Dai Mai when it is not invited. Caution is indicated. The use of Dai Mai is not simply to clear out somebody's closets. Not at all. Very often the unconscious sensation of the ballast Dai Mai can provide is the very security the patient needs. This sense of security is often accompanied by excess weight or accumulation around the middle, around the belt, so it can be tempting to simply drain it out. But Eight Extra pulses are pulses of uneasiness; an inappropriate draining treatment can create tremendous instability and insecurity. The *Mai Jing* is clear that in some treatments the person will heal themselves and in certain circumstances, the patient's condition may significantly worsen. Certain conditions are iatrogenic and arise with the excess intervention of the practitioner. While healing requires change, there must be willingness to change; forcing it is not what healing is about and can result in iatrogenic diseases. A patient must be ready for a Dai Mai treatment in order for it to be warranted.

The Dai Mai pulse reflects these subtleties. It may have an increased uneasiness and an added tightness if it should be consolidated rather than drained. It may feel looser and fuller if it is ready to be drained. The consolidating treatment action is akin to a big deep hug. Draining Dai Mai when it should be consolidated can leave the patient feeling depleted of resources, both emotionally and physically.

BIFURCATED PULSES

A bifurcated pulse is one that feels as though it is split in two. You can feel it traveling to either side of your finger, as though your finger is a kind of median strip. Li Shi Zhen says if the pulse bifurcates at the guan position, Dai Mai is indicated. The split represents the division of Dai Mai into Consolidating Dai Mai and Draining Dai Mai, a departure that occurs at GB-26. Consolidating Dai Mai goes from GB-26 to SP-15 and then to the navel, whereas Draining Dai Mai (the more modern Dai) goes from GB-26 to GB-27 and GB-28. (Li Shi Zhen added LR-13 to the trajectory.) Another interpretation of the split at the guan is the emergence of Bao Mai which runs vertically from Dai Mai.

If a bifurcation is found at the cun position, Yang Qiao Mai is indicated. If at the chi, Yin Qiao Mai is indicated. This is because the Qiao's are the termination of all the Luo Channels. The Luo's have trajectories that connect to the Source, hence the movement of the pulses toward the medial aspect of the wrist. In the chi position, if the pulse is not short, the division into two can be seen to reflect the moving Qi of the Kidneys and its dissemination of Yin and Yang into the two Bladder Shu lines.

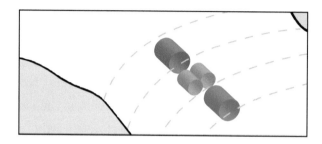

UNILATERAL AND BILATERAL EIGHT EXTRAORDINARY PULSES

If you find Eight Extra pulses on one side, treat the channel/s on that side. (Obviously Ren and Du are not bilateral channels.) Only treat bilaterally if you find the pulses on both wrists. If you choose instead to treat according to gender, the side on which you found the pulse is not important; you would treat on the left in males and on the right in females.

DISPARITY BETWEEN YIN AND YANG

Eight Extraordinary pulses tell us about disparities or imbalances between Yin and Yang. If there are exuberant Yang qualities in the Yuan level causing the deep pulses to be floating, full and big, or floating and long, Yang has gone from the surface to the interior, from the Yang region to the Yin region. The more Yin levels of the pulse (the deep levels) should be relatively quiet.

If there are no pulses on the superficial level and there are also no pulses on the deep level or simply very weak pulses, it means that the Yin quality of the deep pulses has gone to the Yang level, the Wei level. These two scenarios are examples of a disparity between Yin and Yang. They need to be balanced, for example, by building Yin to anchor Yang.

FREQUENTLY ASKED QUESTIONS

1. *Should I roll my fingers over the radial artery to read the Eight Extraordinary Channels more clearly?*

Rolling over the artery is a technique designed to stimulate the Eight Extraordinary pulses, not to diagnose them. Roll your fingers over the artery if you can't feel the Eight Extraordinary pulses at all but want to find them if they are there.

2. *My patient has a Ren Mai pulse but the vibration in the guan position is more prominent than the vibration in the cun or chi positions. What does this mean?*

This means that the treatment should focus on the Ren in the Middle Jiao, especially the intersection of the Ren and the Dai, CV-8.

3. If the Eight Extraordinary pulses are accentuated by turning the wrist on its side, is it better to adopt this position while taking those pulses?

The Eight Extraordinary pulses and the Divergent pulses are more pronounced when the wrist is turned on its side (thumb closest to the ceiling and little finger resting on the table) or if you bend the wrist. However, the technique of using 15 beans of pressure is preferable in eliciting these deep pulses because the entire field of the pulse is open to view in this one stable position. The purpose of mentioning this positioning detail is that the postnatal pulses can be obscured if the wrist is on its side.

4. Why is it important to avoid using the tips of your fingers when taking the pulses?

The tips of the fingers provide too small an area of contact with the skin. Much more information is gleaned by the pads of the fingers. In Eight Extraordinary pulse taking, it is necessary to roll the fingers a little to see how far the pulses extend beyond the cun and the chi positions. This is difficult to do with the reduced contact available when the tips of the fingers are used.

5. When I position my fingers as you describe, the finger on the guan position falls right at the base of the styloid process. Can I really feel the pulse through the bone?

No. Move your finger medially until you feel the pulse clearly.

6. If I find Eight Extraordinary pulses on one side only, are there implications for needling?

Eight Extraordinary pulses are most often found to be one-sided. If the Eight Extraordinary pulses are found on the left side, needle the left side only. If they are found on the right side, needle the right side only. Sun Si Miao taught that the Eight Extras are not needled bilaterally unless the pulse is located bilaterally. Li Shi Zhen considered it disrespectful to Yuan Qi to needle Eight Extraordinary Channels bilaterally.

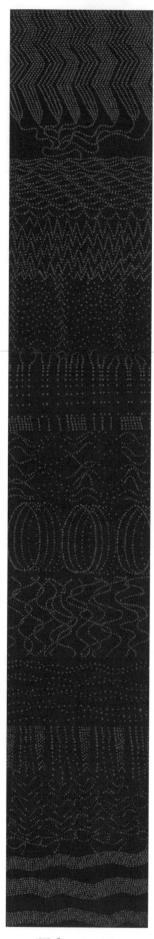

Talisman I

CHAPTER 6
PULSE METHODS IN STEP-BY-STEP PROTOCOLS:
VERY SIMPLE, SIMPLE, AND COMPLEX

PULSE TAKING AND INTENTION

Chapter One of the *Ling Shu* says that when you are treating an individual pay attention to their spirit as well as your own. Do we see them as separate or the same? To see our patient as inseparable from all things is the root of compassion. During the contact that is made while taking the pulse the practitioner imprints on the patient the way in which they can overcome their difficulty. You are imparting healing through the vibration of your intention. Hence one's intention requires a focus generated by one's cultivation. By adopting the view that all is connected, that there is no separation between anyone and anything, it is possible not only to genuinely understand that anything appearing to be negative can be seen as being in the process of being transformed and so can be felt as a deep truth. When you take someone's pulses, you are invoking the Shen and imparting your intentionality. While the client has their individual fire, you as a practitioner are trying to clear the path for their light to shine. Pulse taking is cultivational and not technical.

PULSE TAKING AND INTERACTION

Perhaps the most important factor to keep in mind while engaging the pulses is that the taking of pulses is an interaction. The actions of the practitioner cause the pulse to change. In fact, the practitioner can will the pulse to change, beginning the healing process. The process of taking directional pulses is the same as performing qigong on the pulses. As you press into the Spleen pulse and release the Lung pulse, the act of seeing that connection as active, of imagining its full functioning, will begin to enact that connection. This is what is meant by intention. The task of the practitioner is to provide an environment in which change and healing can occur. If the practitioner is entirely passive and is merely observing, that environment is not being provided. This is not to say that we as practitioners decide what healing means for any one individual. But if a patient asks us to help, we must make a judgment about how that is best done.

Often reporting some of the pulse findings along the way can help tremendously. If you were to find a Small Intestine Sinew pulse, for example, and you reported that to the patient saying, "It seems that your shoulders might be quite tight," the patient will invariably become aware of the tension they are holding there, an awareness they did not have before, and release the shoulders right then and there. Sinew pulses are very easy to change in this way. Various other instances of tightness can be easy to change also. Slippery and wiry qualities are more difficult.

Conversely, some of what we find in the pulses of a given individual might wisely be put aside for another time. If we find in the pulses a history of deep depression but the patient is merely asking for help with dizziness and seems uninterested in getting into a discussion about anything else, we might just focus on the complaint (for example, by nourishing Yin or Blood) and leave aside what seemed to us to be the major finding until an opening is made.

However, we might decide that it is not an infringement to ask the pulses to behave in a different way. This suggestion, offered by our minds, creates effects in the Channels and the Organs which can be immediate and profound. For example, let's say you found that the Stomach pulse was extremely rapid. You could silently ask that pulse to slow down simply by imagining it being slower and by going into a more deeply relaxed state yourself, while remaining physically connected to the pulse. This process, of course, is something every human knows how to do. To calm a baby you take the baby in your arms and make soothing noises while gently rocking, all the while smiling and broadcasting your own calm. Taking the pulses is really no different. We make physical contact with the pulse, make the observations, then create the feeling that what could be different is actually different. We are creating a ripple in consciousness, and consciousness has no boundaries. This is the most important facet of healing. The act of taking the pulse can be as healing or even more healing than the practical treatment itself. Often a patient will report that they already feel much better during pulse taking. This part of the session is golden to the practitioner.

PULSE METHOD

Below you will find a series of pulse methods in increasing complexity, the aim being to offer a plan for students or practitioners new to the approach to jump in and feel comfortable. At first glance the two detailed methods might appear long and laborious. In fact with practice all these steps are performed seamlessly in about five minutes—longer if you are working more as you shift the pulses into a different state, perhaps.

Pulse taking in a nutshell involves determining the height of the pulse (the amount of Yang in that pulse), the width of the pulse (amount of Yin in that pulse), the length of the pulse, whether or not the pulse offers your finger resistance—to determine if it strong, full or empty—the tempo of the pulse and the unique qualities in that position, such as rough, choppy, slippery, scattered, etc.

There are infinite ways to take the pulse. Naturally, every practitioner develops their own style. As with all aspects of Chinese Medicine, a practitioner's style must be personally vivid to them and their patients, and it should harmonize with the Classics.

VERY SIMPLE PULSE METHOD

This method is intended to establish the status of the Spleen Qi and Stomach Fluids with the intention of treating the Spleen and Stomach as the origins of postnatal Qi. It's intended to be used when you have very limited time (if the patient is very late, for example) or if you are beginning to learn pulse diagnosis.

1. Position and approach the patient's pulses as described on page 6.
2. Note any tight pulses between one and three beans of pressure.
3. Move all fingers to the Pulse Neutral position in the right hand. (Cun and guan at the moderate level and chi at the deep level.)
4. Focus attention on the Spleen pulse.
5. Write down one or two textures, describing the Spleen pulse, e.g., slippery, tight.
6. Write down the width of the Spleen pulse.
7. Write down the tempo of the Spleen pulse.
8. Move the Spleen finger down to the Yuan level and write down one or two textures for the Yuan level of the Spleen position.
9. Return to Pulse Neutral.
10. Using the Tilt action, press on the Spleen pulse and, at the same time, release pressure from the Lungs to determine whether the Spleen is ascending to the Lungs.
11. Write down the vector from Spleen to Lungs and mark its status.
12. Note anything outstanding on the right hand and briefly check the left hand pulses first for Sinew pulses. Then look for anything outstanding in the Pulse Neutral position.
13. If you found a Sinew pulse, cup the Sinew indicated. If really short of time, needle the Jing-Well point of the Sinew Channel indicated. Then treat the Spleen as indicated in the pulses.

SIMPLE PULSE METHOD

This method is intended to obtain a broad reading of the pulses without becoming too complex.

For this method I am suggesting what I am calling a Stepped Position where the finger at the cun position is at the Wei level, the finger at the guan position is at the Ying level and the finger at the chi position is at the Yuan level.

1. Position and approach the patient's pulses as described on page 6.
2. At the right wrist, rest the three fingers at one bean of pressure and note the location of the Sinew pulses if any.
3. Move all fingers to the Stepped Position. Lift each finger gradually to establish the height of Yang.
4. Move all fingers back to the Stepped Position. While in the Stepped Position, examine the width of the pulses at the cun, guan and chi positions.
5. While in the Stepped Position, measure the tempo of the pulses at the cun, guan and chi positions.
6. While in the Stepped Position, note the texture of the pulses at the cun, guan and chi positions.
7. Assume Pulse Neutral position. Using the tilt action, determine whether the Spleen is ascending Qi to the Lungs. Add a little pressure to the Spleen pulse while releasing pressure from the Lungs.
8. Check to see whether the Lungs disperse.
9. Move to the left wrist.
10. At the left wrist, rest the three fingers at one bean of pressure and note the location of the Sinew pulses if any.
11. Move all fingers to the Stepped Position. Lift each finger gradually to establish the height of Yang and chart them.
12. Move all fingers back to the Stepped Position. While in the Stepped Position, examine the width of the pulses at the cun, guan and chi positions and chart them.
13. While in the Stepped Position, measure the tempo of the pulses at the cun, guan and chi positions and chart them.
14. While in the Stepped Position, note the texture of the pulses at the cun, guan and chi positions and chart them.
15. Assume Pulse Neutral position. Using the tilt action, determine whether the Liver is ascending Blood to the Heart. Add a little pressure to the Liver pulse while releasing pressure from the Heart position.
16. Check to see whether the Heart disperses by gradually releasing pressure from it.
17. Assume Pulse Neutral position. Using the tilt action, determine whether the Liver is sharing its Blood with the Kidneys. Add a little pressure to the Liver while releasing a little pressure from the Kidneys.
18. Note any blockages if you notice them. See Inter-Jiao Blockages, page 97.
19. Note anything else outstanding.

Below you will find two detailed methods, one focusing on directional pulses and one focused on probing pulses. Neither is superior. The directional focus is my preference, but that's probably simply because I really enjoy examining directionality. It seems to offer a greater opportunity for dialogue with the pulses. It also feels (to me) easier to perform qigong on the pulses, to train the connections between organs and to train organ function. Of course probing pulses offer the same dialogue with the practitioner; all this is merely personal preference. After practicing these methods you'll find your own balance between them.

COMPLEX PULSE METHOD FOCUSING ON DIRECTIONALITY

Detailed background information for this method is in Chapter 4.

While performing this method, watch for the following things at all times:

Note inter-Jiao blockages. These show as a swelling between the cun and guan or the guan and chi.

They also show during a tilt action when the pulse that you are pressing down on becomes larger while the receiving pulse does not pop.

At any time, be aware if the pulse you are feeling begins to move laterally from side to side. This is a moving pulse and is telling you that the most appropriate treatment is likely to be a Divergent or Eight Extraordinary Channel treatment. If you practice these channels, immediately examine the Divergent and Eight Extraordinary pulses.

RIGHT SIDE

1. Position and approach the patient's pulses as described on page 6.
2. Rest the three fingers on the right wrist at one bean of pressure. Move the fingers between one and three beans of pressure.
3. Write down the location of any Sinew Pulse present.
4. If there is a Sinew pulse present, press a little deeper (perhaps three beans deeper) and see whether there are resources present to push the external pathogenic factor (EPF) out of the Sinew Channel. Right under the (tight) Sinew pulse there must be both width and upward pressure in the pulse to enable that to happen. The width tells us whether there are sufficient fluids available to carry the pathogen out. The upward pressure tells us whether sufficient Wei Qi is available to push the pathogen out. One of these factors is likely out of balance; otherwise the body would have eradicated the pathogen and wouldn't be showing a Sinew pulse.

5. Write down the status of Fluids and Qi in that location by noting the width of the pulse and whether the pulse is pushing upward.

6. Move all fingers to the Pulse Neutral position. (Cun and guan at the moderate level and chi at the deep level.)

7. Focus attention on the Spleen pulse.

8. Write down one or two textures, describing the Spleen pulse.

9. Note the width of the Spleen pulse.

10. Note the tempo of the Spleen pulse.

11. If the length of the Spleen pulse is unusual, note it.

12. Move the Spleen finger down to the Yuan level and note whether the Spleen pulse offers you resistance as you make that movement.

13. Write down one or two textures for the Yuan level of the Spleen position.

14. Focus on the Lung pulse.

15. Write down one or two textures, describing the Lung pulse.

16. Note the width of the Lung pulse.

17. Note the tempo of the Lung pulse.

18. If the length of the Lung pulse is unusual, note it.

19. Move the Lung finger down to the Yuan level and note whether the Lung pulse offers you resistance as you make that movement.

20. Write down one or two textures for the Yuan level of the Lung position.

21. As slowly as possible, release pressure from the Lung pulse.

22. Draw the vector showing the degree to which it disperses.

23. Return to Pulse Neutral.

24. Using the Tilt action, press on the Spleen pulse and at the same time, release pressure from the Lungs to determine whether the Spleen is ascending to the Lungs.

25. Write down the vector from Spleen to Lungs and mark its status.

26. Return to Pulse Neutral.

27. Focus on the Kidney Yang pulse.

28. Write down one or two textures, describing the Kidney Yang pulse.

29. Note the width of the Kidney Yang pulse.

30. Note the tempo of the Kidney Yang pulse.

31. If the length of the Kidney Yang pulse is unusual, note it.

32. As slowly as possible, release pressure from the Kidney Yang pulse.

33. Note whether the pulse is present above the Yuan level and the location of such a pulse.

34. Return to Pulse Neutral.

35. Using the Tilt action, add a tiny amount of pressure to the Stomach pulse and release a tiny amount of pressure from the Kidney Yang pulse, to determine whether the

Stomach descends.

36. Draw the vector from Stomach to Kidney and mark its status.

37. Return to Pulse Neutral.

38. Using the Tilt action, add a tiny amount of pressure to the Lung pulse and release a tiny amount of pressure from the Kidney Yang pulse, to determine whether the Lungs descend.

39. Draw the vector from Lungs to Kidneys and mark its status.

40. Gently remove your hand.

41. Change sides.

LEFT SIDE

1. Rest the three fingers on the left wrist at one bean of pressure. Move the fingers between one and three beans of pressure.

2. Write down the location of any Sinew Pulse present.

3. If there is a Sinew pulse present, press a little deeper (perhaps three beans deeper) and see whether there are resources present to push the external pathogenic factor (EPF) out of the Sinew Channel. Right under the (tight) Sinew pulse there must be both width and pressure upward in the pulse to enable that to happen. The width tells us the complement of fluids available to carry the pathogen out, and the pressure upward tells us whether sufficient Wei Qi is available to push the pathogen out. One of these factors is likely out of balance; otherwise the body would have eradicated it.

4. Move all fingers to the Pulse Neutral position. (Cun and guan at the moderate level and chi at the deep level.)

5. Focus attention on the Liver pulse.

6. Write down one or two textures, describing the Liver pulse.

7. Note the width of the Liver pulse.

8. Note the tempo of the Liver pulse.

9. If the length of the Liver pulse is unusual, note it.

10. Move the Liver finger down to the Yuan level and note whether the Liver pulse offers you resistance as you make that movement.

11. Write down one or two textures for the Yuan level of the Liver position.

12. Focus on the Heart pulse.

13. Write down one or two textures, describing the Heart pulse.

14. Note the width of the Heart pulse.

15. Note the tempo of the Heart pulse.

16. If the length of the Heart pulse is unusual, note it.

17. Move the Heart finger down to the Yuan level and note whether the Heart pulse offers you resistance as you make that movement.

18. Write down one or two textures for the Yuan level of the Heart position.
19. As slowly as possible, release pressure from the Heart pulse.
20. Draw the vector showing the degree to which it disperses.
21. Return to Pulse Neutral.
22. Using the Tilt action, press on the Liver pulse and at the same time release pressure from the Heart to determine whether Liver Blood is ascending to the Heart.
23. Write down the vector from Liver to Heart and mark its status.
24. Return to Pulse Neutral.
25. Focus on the Kidney Yin pulse.
26. Write down one or two textures, describing the Kidney Yin pulse.
27. Note the width of the Kidney Yin pulse.
28. Note the tempo of the Kidney Yin pulse.
29. If the length of the Kidney Yin pulse is unusual, note it.
30. Using the Tilt action, add a tiny amount of pressure to the Liver pulse and release a tiny amount of pressure from the Kidney pulse, to determine whether Liver Blood is nourishing Kidney Yin. (If it is not, see if Kidney Yin is breaking down to make Liver Blood by pressing down on the Kidney and releasing from the Liver.)
31. Draw the vector from Liver to Kidney and mark its status.
32. Return to Pulse Neutral.
33. Using the Tilt action, add a tiny amount of pressure to the Heart pulse and release a tiny amount of pressure from the Kidney pulse, to determine whether the Heart communicates to the Kidneys.
34. Draw the vector from Heart to Kidney and mark its status.
35. Return to Pulse Neutral.
36. Using the Tilt action, add a tiny amount of pressure to the Kidney pulse and release a tiny amount of pressure from the Heart pulse, to determine whether the Kidney communicates to the Heart.
37. Draw the vector from Kidney to Heart and mark its status.
38. Return to Pulse Neutral.
39. Gently remove your hand.
(Optional) Examine the Divergent and Eight Extra pulses.

COMPLEX PULSE METHOD FOCUSING ON PROBING PULSES
Detailed background information for this method is in Chapter 3.

While performing this method, be aware of the following things at all times:
Throughout this method, there must be pressure applied to the cun, guan and chi, regardless of whether a position is the focus of attention or not. If pressure is not applied to all three

positions—even as moving pressure is applied to only one—the readings will not be accurate since the pressure at the two idle positions simulates the systemic interactions of the matrix of Qi. To take pulses with one or two fingers only is to examine the organ out of the context of its connections to any other organ and gives a false view of that organ.

Note inter-Jiao blockages. These show as a swelling between the cun and guan or the guan and chi.

At any time, be aware if the pulse you are feeling begins to move laterally from side to side. This is a moving pulse and is telling you that the most appropriate treatment is likely to be a Divergent or Eight Extra Channel treatment. If you practice these channels, proceed at this point to examine the Divergent and Eight Extra pulses.

1. Rest your fingers at between one and three beans of pressure and note the location of any Sinew pulses.
2. Assume Pulse Neutral position at the right hand.

RIGHT GUAN POSITION

3. Focus on the moderate level of the guan position, the Spleen pulse. Note the width, length, tempo and texture of the moderate level. It's natural for the Spleen to be very slightly slippery only in the moderate level. If the Spleen has integrity at its borders and is robust and buoyant, it is functioning well to temper thinking and resolve problems—it's able to control the Mind. It is able to transform and transport food; it can extract Qi from food. It can manage Blood.

4. Allow your guan finger to rise to the superficial level. Note the width, length, tempo and texture. Press slowly back down into the moderate level. If the pulse becomes slightly bigger, the Stomach is able to descend Qi to the rest of the digestive tract.

5. Move your guan finger from the moderate to the deep level. Note the width, length, tempo and texture. If the pulse becomes slightly stronger, the Spleen is able to perform its ascending functions, notably the ascension of Kidney Yang to the Stomach. It is able also to ascend pure thin fluids to the sensory orifices and to bring the red substance up to the Heart to finalize the production of Blood. If it is nice and wide, it is able to produce Gu Qi (Qi and Blood). If there is no slipperiness here, the Spleen is meeting the demands of the body in resolving Damp and controlling the four limbs.

6. If the strength of the sensation in pressing from superficial to moderate matches the sensation of pressing from moderate to deep, the Stomach and Spleen are harmonized.

7. Return to Pulse Neutral.

RIGHT CUN POSITION

8. Focus on the moderate level of the cun position, the Lung pulse. Note the width, length, tempo and texture of the moderate level. If strong, the origin of Qi is strong. If

strong and clear of pathology, the Lungs are able to rectify Qi.

9. Slowly release pressure on the Lung pulse. It should float with a steady consistent pressure to the Wei level. This confirms that the Lungs can let go of Qi during respiration, that they can disperse Qi. If dispersion is good between the moderate and superficial levels they can move Blood. The patient is able to let go and accept life.

10. Press back very slightly into the superficial level of the Lung pulse. Note the width, length, tempo and texture of the superficial level. If adequately wide, the Lungs are able to move mediumship and are getting Fluids from the Stomach.

11. Press down into the deep level of the Lung pulse. Note the width, length, tempo and texture of the deep level. The Lung pulse should become stronger and fuller at the deep level. This shows the Lungs are able to descend Qi.

12. Be sure to have noted any slippery, wiry, tight or beady pulses. These indicate key pathologies of the Lungs.

13. Return to Pulse Neutral.

RIGHT CHI POSITION

14. Focus on the deep level of the chi position, the Kidney Yang pulse. Note the width, length, tempo and texture of the deep level. It should be strong. It should be faster than its Yin partner which we have yet to look at. This indicates that the Kidneys are producing warmth, movement and enthusiasm for life and that they are able to disseminate Jing to the Bladder Shu points, maintaining the minute-to-minute functioning of the organs. If the pulse feels solidly anchored in the deep level, the Will is strong. The lower orifices can be controlled. A rapid pulse on the right chi may not be pathological; it might simply be reflecting enthusiasm for life. A slightly tight Kidney Yang pulse may be acting to prevent leakage. A soft one may be present if the patient is in a deeply relaxed state. If the pulse is wide, the Kidneys can provide the moving energy for Triple Heater function and the regulation of the waterways, the production of Jing-Essence and Qi.

15. Press more deeply into the deep level. If the pulse becomes stronger, the patient is able to navigate their own destiny. They can be true to themselves. The patient also has secure Jing-Essence; structure can be maintained.

16. Allow your finger to move upward from the deep to the moderate level. The pulse should follow you to the cusp of the deep and moderate levels and remain strong as it does so. If it does, the Kidneys are providing the Yang Qi to the Triple Heater to enable the dissemination of Jing to the Bladder Shu points, which in turn transport that Jing to the organs for the expression of life. The pulse should not follow your finger into the moderate level. If it does, there is either insufficient Qi to hold Yin down, or insufficient Yin to hold down in the first place. This will become clear when you examine the width of the left Kidney pulse, a pulse that should also be contained in the deep level. If the pulse does rise to the moderate level, note its qualities.

17. Slowly move from around nine beans of pressure and press back into the deep level of the chi, to 15 beans. As you are making this journey, note whether the pulse becomes steadily stronger. If it does, the Kidneys are able to receive Qi from the Lungs and Stomach if it is offered (if the Lungs and Stomach are descending their Qi).

18. Make special note of the presence of pathological qualities of the Kidneys. That is, note if the pulse is weak, slow, tight, too rapid, wiry, scattered, floating beyond the Yuan level or a combination of any of the above.

19. Return to Pulse Neutral.

MOVE TO THE LEFT WRIST.

20. Rest your fingers at between one and three beans of pressure and note the location of any Sinew pulses.

21. Assume Pulse Neutral position at the left hand.

LEFT GUAN POSITION

22. Focus on the moderate level of the guan position, the Liver pulse. Note the width, length, tempo and texture of the moderate level. It is normal for the Liver pulse to be slightly tight at the moderate level, especially between six and nine beans. If slightly tight, the Liver is able to store Blood, contain the Hun, store memory, and is able to plan and hold that plan. Sometimes it is tighter in women because its principal function is to gather and store Blood. It should not be wiry, as that would indicate stagnation.

23. Slowly decrease pressure on the guan position, allowing it to go up into the superficial level of the pulse. If the pulse moves up with you, the Liver is able to ascend Qi. It can bring its Blood up to the Heart to engender Heart Qi. There is sufficient Liver Blood for the realization of one's destiny or life's purpose. There are resources for achievement. If it becomes apparent that the pulse is wide as you are allowing the pulse to go up, Liver Blood is able to engender Heart Blood. The Liver is able to bring Blood to the Sinews. Check that the Liver pulse can follow you up to three beans of pressure. If so, the Liver can deliver Blood to the brain and can open to the eyes, enlivening them and generating interest in life. Note the width, length, tempo and texture of the superficial level.

24. Return to the moderate level. Slowly increase pressure on the guan position, pressing it into the deep level. If the pulse responds by pushing against your finger as you increase the pressure on it as you reach the cusp of the moderate and deep levels, the Liver is able to descend Blood to the Lower Jiao. Liver Blood is able to nourish Yin and Jing-Essence. If you found that the Liver followed your finger in the previous step and offered resistance to your finger during this current step, the Liver is able to regulate Qi. It is able to spread Qi through both Yin and Yang Sinews, which in turn control all the smooth muscle and the exterior. As long as it is able to maintain integrity in the moderate level, it is normal to find that the Liver pulse softens slightly as you reach the

deep level. This indicates the Liver is able to discharge its Dampness by temporarily creating loose stools.

25. Press deeper, beyond 12 beans into the Liver pulse. Note the width, length, tempo and texture of the deep level. Go slowly to 14 beans of pressure (just before the occlusion of blood in the radial artery). As you approach 14 beans, the pulse may feel as though it is disintegrating. This demonstrates that the Liver can break up Blood to nourish the Essence. The Liver softens the Blood so that it can become Jing. If the pulse at this level is plentiful, the Liver can nourish the structure, hair, skin and nails. It can also share enough Blood with the Kidneys to foster self-worth. If, as you move through the juncture of the moderate and deep levels, you feel that the pulse is wide and then softens into a wide pulse at the deep level, and especially if there is a feeling of real density yet softening at the deep level, the Liver is able to provide ample Blood to nourish Kidney Yin. This is a marker of fertility.

26. Make special note of qualities that show pathology in the Liver. The pulse should not be thin as it is pressed more deeply, especially when pressed beyond 12 beans. The Liver pulse should not scatter. That indicates Wind in the Liver. To store Blood there must be Qi at the Liver position; it cannot be weak, empty, frail or minute. A weak Liver pulse indicates that there is insufficient Qi to store Blood and so Liver Blood cannot be nourishing the Kidneys to support Jing-Essence. If the Liver pulse is weak on the deep level, the Liver hasn't enough Qi to bring that Blood to support the Essence and the structure. And most of all, the Liver cannot be wiry at all. A stagnated Liver prevents the smooth flow of Qi, oppresses the diaphragm and can stymy all other Liver functions including storing Blood. A wiry or thin Liver pulse indicates that the Liver cannot nourish the Heart and Kidneys. A Wiry quality is often a result of long-term Cold. Moxa on LR-12 breaks up Cold in the Liver. Wiry should not be confused with tight, which is not necessarily pathological. A rapid Liver pulse will elevate Heat in the Heart and Blood. A slow Liver pulse shows that the Liver is stagnating Blood. The Liver pulse should not float to, or be full at the superficial level. A slippery Liver pulse indicates an imbalance between the Liver and the Spleen. Treat the Spleen since the Spleen is not controlling Damp.

27. Return to Pulse Neutral.

LEFT CUN

28. Focus on the moderate level of the cun position, the Heart pulse. Note the width, length, tempo and texture of the moderate level. It is normal for the Heart to have Yang qualities, to be strong and to have an excited feeling about it. If the pulse is strong at the moderate level, the Heart is able to invigorate Blood.

29. Lift your finger a small amount, very slowly. The pulse should feel full and follow you up. At best, it will become fuller as it follows you. This means that there is enough Blood

for the conduction of experiences, excitement and interaction. This is what the Heart seeks but it needs to conduct Blood to do so. There is enough Blood to nourish the Shen because the Heart is able to be curious and excited. The pulse might scatter as it moves upward into the superficial level. This means that Heart Blood is reaching the tongue to express and share joy and excitement. At the superficial level, and only at that level, there might be a very slight tight quality. This is the action of the Shen being held in place and is not pathological. Note the width, length, tempo and texture of the superficial level. Note that you might find that the Heart pulse has moved up to the superficial level because the patient is delighted to find that you are interested in them. A Heart-to-Heart conversation that is part of an acupuncture treatment encounter, moves the Heart.

30. Press down on the pulse, nearing the Yuan level. The pulse should feel very relaxed during that transit. This means that there is enough Blood for the the full emanation of love. There is enough Blood to carry the destiny contained in the Jing-Essence. As you settle your finger into the deep level (the retreat of the Shen) the pulse should continue to be very relaxed, even gentle and soft. This means the Kidneys are receiving the Yang Qi from the Heart and they are able to calm the Shen; the Shen is anchored. If the pulse at the deep level is not relaxed, the patient is unable to calm themselves or they have insomnia, or both. Note the width, length, tempo and texture of the deep level.

31. Note the presence of any qualities you found at any depth that are pathological to the Heart. A wiry Heart pulse indicates either that the Heart is constrained by Dampness or Phlegm or that the patient is knowingly or unknowingly agreeing to a limitation being placed on the amount of joy their Heart is allowed to express. A tight pulse shows obstruction or stagnation in the Heart, except at the superficial level. A rapid Heart pulse is showing that there is too much excitement, causing Heat. If the Heart becomes rapid as it scatters, there is too much stimulation. An urgent Heart pulse can indicate the presence of an entity. A slippery Heart pulse indicates Phlegm in the gut. The phlegm should have been expectorated by the Lungs but the Lungs might have been weak or are currently weak. The Heart should have no Yin factors. Yin factors (Damp and Phlegm) hamper its freedom.

32. Return to Pulse Neutral.

LEFT CHI POSITION

33. Focus on the deep level of the chi position, the Kidney Yin pulse. Note the width, length, tempo and texture of the deep level. It should feel strong, full and slightly tight, as their principal function is to conserve Jing-Essence and to optimize the availability of Jing for the carrying out of one's destiny. Classically, this is known as the stone pulse as it feels so heavy. It should be slower than its right hand counterpart. This is not to be confused with Cold. Jing is precious and is to be conserved. It is naturally slow and

dense.

34. Slowly release pressure on the Kidney pulse at the deep level. The pulse should follow your finger to the cusp of the moderate level and still feel strong.

35. Slowly release pressure further. The pulse should not follow you into the moderate level. It certainly should not follow you into the superficial level.

(Optional) Examine the Divergent and Eight Extra pulses.

CHAPTER 7

DIAGNOSIS AND TREATMENT PRINCIPLES

Diagnoses are made based on the observations of the five parameters: height, width, length, tempo and texture, along with either or both directional and probing pulses, keeping the functions of the organs in mind the entire time.

The beauty of this detailed way of looking at the pulses is that you can see whether the weakness perceived in an organ pulse is actually reflecting weakness in that organ, or whether the organ is not being supplied with Qi or mediumship by the organ that has that responsibility. Therefore, be careful about diagnosing weakness in any organ. If your diagnosis is of weakness of an organ that is not in fact weak, the treatment may produce no results.

Keep in mind the following:
- The Lung pulse might appear weak if the Spleen is not ascending its Qi to the Lungs. Check that Spleen Qi is ascending to the Lungs before declaring the Lungs weak. If the Spleen is not ascending Qi, treat the ascending function of the Spleen and check the Lung pulse again.
- The Lung pulse might appear weak if the Kidneys are deficient in Qi. If the Kidneys are weak, tonify Kidney Qi and take the pulse again to see if the Lungs respond.
- The Lung pulse might appear weak if the Spleen is not ascending Qi from the Kidneys to the Spleen.
- The Lungs might appear weak if there is a diaphragmatic blockage, if there is Damp in the Spleen, if there are wiry pulses in the guan position on either side, etc.
- The Lungs might appear weak if there is a deficiency of Stomach Fluids. Nourish Stomach Fluids and check the pulse again.
- The Heart may appear weak if it is not receiving Blood from the Liver. The Spleen is responsible for that ascension. Before declaring the Heart weak, nourish Liver Blood and check the Heart pulse again. (There is no such thing as the tonification of Heart Qi. Heart Qi and Heart Blood come solely from the Blood of the Liver, ascended to the Heart by the Spleen.)
- Any pulse can appear tight if it is trying to conserve the mediumship related to it. The Liver can be tight (normally, actually) as it stores Blood, the Spleen pulse can be tight if the Stomach is trying to reserve Fluids, the Kidneys can be tight if they are trying to conserve Jing.

159

If you see clearly where the pathology is coming from in the pulses and make your diagnosis based on that, you will truly treat the root of the condition. Use your knowledge of point function to create the changes described. (On page 96 I have included some basic treatment ideas for some of these pathologies below, to help students get started.) I've respectfully and deliberately not offered treatment protocols here; that's where acupuncture becomes an art as much as it is a science. Choosing the right points for the individual requires knowledge and a feel for the points. Knowledge of point function is a basic part of all acupuncturists' education, fortunately.

DIAGNOSIS FOR VERY SIMPLE PULSE METHOD (SAMPLE)
Checklist:
- Where are the excesses and deficiencies?
- Did the Spleen ascend?

Given all your observations in the method above, your diagnosis might include one or more of the following, or other observations.

- Wind in the _____ Sinew Channel, if you found a superficial, tight pulse.
- _____ (Damp, Cold, Damp-Heat, Qi deficiency, etc.) in the Spleen.
- Deficiency of Stomach Fluids.
- Failure of the Spleen to ascend Qi.

TREATMENT PRINCIPLES FOR VERY SIMPLE PULSE METHOD (SAMPLE)
Your treatment principles might include one or more of the following, or others.

- Release the _____ Sinew Channel.
- Tonify Spleen Qi, Resolve Damp or Damp-Heat or Cold in the Spleen.
- Nourish Stomach Fluids.
- Ascend Spleen Qi.

DIAGNOSIS FOR SIMPLE PULSE METHOD
Checklist:
- Where are the excesses and deficiencies?
- In the cun position, did you feel a pulse at the Wei level? Did it stand out in any way? Was the width notable? Was the length notable? Was the tempo notable? Did it have a notable texture?
- In the guan position, did you feel a pulse at the Ying level? Did it stand out in any

way? Was the width notable? Was the length notable? Was the tempo notable? Did it have a notable texture?

- In the chi position, did you feel a pulse at the Yuan level? Did it stand out in any way? Was the width notable? Was the length notable? Was the tempo notable? Did it have a notable texture?

Given all your observations in the method, your diagnosis might include one or more of the following, or other observations.

- Wind in the _____ Sinew Channel, if you found a superficial, tight pulse.
- _____ (Cold, Heat, Damp, Damp-Heat, Qi deficiency, Heat, Wind, etc.) in the _____ (organ).
- Deficiency of _____ (Fluids, Blood, Jing).
- Failure of the _____ to _____.

TREATMENT PRINCIPLES FOR SIMPLE PULSE METHOD

Your treatment principles might include one or more of the following, or others.

- Nourish/Tonify _____ (Jin-Thin Fluids, Blood, Qi, Ye-Thick Fluids, Jing.)
- Ascend/Descend/Course/Disperse _____ (name of organ).

DIAGNOSIS FOR EITHER OF THE COMPLEX PULSE METHODS

Checklist:

- Where are the excesses and deficiencies that stood out to you?
- In any position (cun, guan or chi), at any of the three depths (superficial, moderate or deep), did you find any outstanding qualities of the five parameters (height, width, length, tempo or texture)
- Did you find any of the vectors missing? (Was the directionality of each organ demonstrated in the pulses as you performed the tilts and releases?)
- Did you notice any inter-Jiao blockages?
- Did you notice any of the pulses becoming moving pulses?
- Look at your notation of blockages and your arrows of directionality. Satisfy yourself about whether tight pulses indicate a blockage or whether the tightness is the response of the body to a deficient humor. Using the arrows, explain why the various media (Fluids and Qi) are excess or deficient. This explanation will become part of your diagnosis.

Given all your observations in the method, your diagnosis might include one or more of the following, or other observations.

- Wind-Cold/Heat/Damp in the _____ Sinew Channel, if you found a superficial, tight pulse.
- _____ (Cold, Heat, Damp, Damp-Heat, Qi deficiency, Heat, Wind, etc.) in the _____ (organ).
- Deficiency of _____ (Fluids, Blood, Jing). Or Excesses.
- Failure of _____ (organ/Qi) to generate or nourish: Blood/Qi/Wei/Ying/Jing
- Blockage between ____ and _____ or: failure of _____ to communicate with _____.
- Any other findings.

TREATMENT PRINCIPLES FOR EITHER OF THE COMPLEX PULSE METHODS

Your treatment principles might include one or more of the following, or others.

- Release the _____ Sinew.
- Nourish/Tonify _____ (Jin-Thin Fluids, Blood, Qi, Ye-Thick Fluids, Jing.)
- Ascend/Descend/Course/Disperse/Resolve/Dissolve/Rectify, etc. _____ .
- If you noticed blockages, release them first, and then re-check the pulses to make sure your diagnosis is still valid.
- If you noticed moving pulses, examine the Eight Extra and or the Divergent pulses.

DIAGNOSIS NOT BASED ON PULSES

The Luo Channels are diagnosed by observation. The main reason to take pulses if you have already decided to treat the Luo Channels is that it helps you understand how best to nourish Blood after the treatment if that becomes necessary. Generally, however, simple regulation of Blood using even technique one point proximal to the He-Sea point is perfectly adequate.

CHAPTER 8

PULSE DIAGNOSIS AND DIET

Andrew Sterman
From his book *The Language Food Speaks*, 2017

The branch of Chinese Medicine known as Dietary Therapy distinguishes itself from other types of dietary advice by, like acupuncture and Chinese herbal medicine, relying fully upon pulse and tongue diagnosis. The emphasis is utterly upon individual health needs and matching foods (and cooking methods) precisely to the individual, always within a well-formed strategy. Properly conceived and implemented, dietary therapy can be a stand-alone therapeutic modality, and at the very least every acupuncture or herbal patient should be offered dietary advice to maximize the effectiveness of each session.

As a full practice in its own right, dietary therapy is a lifelong study requiring years of study and practice to bring to a high level. In the context of a pulse diagnosis manual, however, there are many important associations to make. This section is intended as an invitation to integrate dietary therapy very closely with acupuncture or herbal treatments.

TO ENGENDER OR ELICIT THE PULSE

The pulses could be deep in the flesh or hard to find due to a deficiency of Fluids or of Yang Qi, or as a sign of depression.

To build fluids, nourish Stomach Yin with steamed rice or steamed millet. In the morning, congee or other wet breakfasts (oatmeal, millet porridge, cream of wheat [if well tolerated], polenta, quinoa, etc.) can quickly make an enormous difference. Take care with the overuse of the sticky grains (wheat, short grain rices and oats) as they can create Dampness.

To build Kidney Yin to support digestion at a deeper level, use nuts. Those with a Kidney affinity are walnuts, cashews and peanuts. Nuts for the Middle Jiao are pecans, hazelnuts, macadamia, and Brazil nuts.

To move Yang Qi to the exterior (and bring the pulses with it, similar to the Engender Pulse Decoction in herbal medicine), choose vegetables that have an upward directionality (asparagus) and that spread Qi (collard, kale, chard). Then use spices to bring those qualities to the exterior: cinnamon, ginger, turmeric, parsley, thyme, rosemary, oregano, etc. All spices move Yang Qi. Select spices according to what is appropriate and tolerable for the patient; some spices are too warming for some people and others stimulate through heat and irritation (garlic, onion, hot chili peppers). Nightshades such as tomatoes also invigorate Yang Qi and invigorate Blood, helping to bring pulses to the fore, but be mindful of their appropriateness as they invigorate Yang Qi through irritation. In any case, dietary advice for the patient to help engender the pulse is not a long-term measure.

Fruits also help move Yang Qi to the exterior (fruits are the Yang expression of their tree or plant). Tart or sour fruits, however, tend to be astringent and restraining. Reserve their use for banking Blood while using gently sweet fruits to engender the pulse.

WIDTH AT THE THREE LEVELS OF THE PULSE

Before the historical emphasis on Zang-Fu organs in Chinese Medicine, humors were the focus, or more specifically, the three levels of Qi: Wei Qi, Ying Qi and Yuan Qi. A well-balanced diet for maintenance naturally focuses on the Ying-Nutritive Qi level, which in turn nourishes all aspects of body energetics. For therapeutic purposes, foods can be selected to work more specifically with Wei and Yuan Qi.

Width at the Wei Level indicates the status of Jin-Thin fluids. If deficient, nourish Stomach Yin with steamed grains and porridges (especially as morning food, during the time of the Stomach and Spleen/Pancreas).

Width at the Ying Level indicates relative sufficiency of Blood. Again, grains are very important for building blood, since Stomach Fluids are the origin of Blood. The most moistening grains are millet, rice (short or medium grain), oats, barley and corn. Dark green vegetables provide nutrients and energetics essential for building blood. Red kale, red cabbage and red chard, in keeping with the law of signature, have stood the test of time for aiding with building Blood. Animal food is not essential but makes Blood building vastly easier for most people. Foods of note are beef and bison, particularly in soup or stews. Eggs help build Blood, particularly in soup (egg drop soup or eggs with rice congee). Root vegetables and tubers strengthen the Spleen and help build Blood (beets, sweet potatoes). Berries (blueberries, raspberries, goji berries) help build and bank Blood. Certain beans help build Blood, especially adzuki beans. While building Blood, it is essential to invigorate Blood (with use of spices, vegetables or fruits, see above) and then to bank Blood. Help store Blood that is being built with sour or tart foods. Some, such as goji berries or raspberries, include that tart flavor, helping to build and bank Blood concurrently.

Width at the Yuan Level indicates the status of Ye-Thick Fluids including hormones. Nourish the Yuan Level if needed with shellfish (clams, mussels, oysters, abalone, etc.), seaweed, mushrooms, nuts and seeds (especially sesame seeds). Hydration is key here as well, but here hydration includes not only water fluids but also fats, including nut oils and animal fats (butter, for example). Bone broths nourish at this level.

SLIPPERY OR LONG PULSES

Reduce foods that easily cause Dampness (sugar, cheese, gluten, alcohol), advise to eat at more regular times and with less worry (to allow the Spleen/Pancreas to function better) and increase Damp draining foods (mushrooms, barley, bitter greens, etc.) Any reduction of Dampness or Phlegm will automatically strengthen the Spleen/Pancreas's ability to hold things in their boundaries, which in turn will be reflected by the pulses not overflowing their normal positions.

RAPID PULSES

Rapid pulses can have many causes and therefore include several dietary considerations. The misuse of hot spices could be involved, especially garlic, onions, hot peppers, as well as coffee or chocolate. Nightshades tend to invigorate the Blood through irritation, potentially bringing too much Heat to the Blood, showing as rapid pulses. Protein is warming and stimulates Stomach Fire for proper digestion; too much protein may be a cause of rapid pulses. Stagnation could be a cause of Heat as the body tries to move the stagnation. The timing of eating and sleeping could be involved. The Stomach likes to be quiet during sleep. Eating late at night causes Heat to rise in the Stomach, eventually spreading. The emotions need to be considered. Eating when emotionally upset disturbs digestion. Eating to calm emotional upset is very common. A strategy to resolve that habit is very important.

In the simplest strategy, Heat is cleared and cooled (cooling without clearing can trap heat internally). An easy dish to clear and cool is made by lightly cooking mung sprouts. Sauté for only one or two minutes with ginger and scallion, a splash of good quality oil and pinch of salt. (Avoid chicken stock—common in restaurant cooking—because it tends to be very warming.) Sprouts are very cooling and also clearing; the ginger and scallion will increase movement of fluids and gently protect digestion from the cooling energy of the sprouts. A side dish is eaten two or three times a day for a few days. If progress is not apparent in the pulses, a more advanced strategy may be needed.

Specific foods can be fine-tuned to the location of the rapid pulse. Congee and other grain porridges nourish Stomach Yin, providing fluids necessary for clearing. Small beans clear; select by color for Zang Fu association. Bitter greens are cooling and clearing, as are, for that matter, most vegetarian meals that avoid high fat or hot spices. A more conceptual approach using elemental relationships is also common: drain overstimulation of one organ by reducing stimulation to its Mother Element and/or increasing focus on its Child Element.

SLOW PULSES

If pulses are slow, indicating Cold, warming spices may be helpful, particularly ginger and turmeric. All food should be cooked. Advise the individual to abstain from all raw or cold food, at least as an experiment for a limited time. This includes salads, juices, smoothies, ice cream, raw fruit and vegetables. Check the Lung and Heart pulses for dispersion; depression may be involved.

TEXTURES

It is never appropriate to say, "Given that you have this pulse, you must eat that food." Rather, food associations are meant as possibilities to represent ways of thinking. As with famous teaching formulas in herbal medicine, it is expected that the clinician will use the suggestions as anchors for memory and adapt according to the patient's individual presentations (and with diet, very importantly, their likes, dislikes, sensitivities and cultural background).

1. **Weak, Insufficient, Frail, Minute** Use Yang foods (meat, chicken, dairy, large beans, asparagus). Keep in mind that digestive capacity will be weak, so strong foods may be overly taxing. Then, use foods that stimulate appetite and prepare Stomach Fire for digestion/assimilation (true appetizers): pickles/brined food, fermented foods, small sips of plum wine or sherry, bitter foods (including olives and artichokes, which are often brined) or root vegetables for descension (carrots, beets).
2. **Exuberant, Full** The diet may be working well. If there is excess Yang, avoid foods that are very Yang or very moving (see Rapid pulses, above).
3. **Rapid** Reduce Heat in diet (see Rapid Pulses, above).
4. **Slow** Reduce Cold and Damp in diet (see Slow pulses, above).
5. **Tight** If pathological, use warming spices and leafy green vegetables. If physiological response (healthy), nourish the deficient humor.
6. **Wiry, Bowstring** Invigorate and relax Yang. Eliminate raw foods; all foods should be cooked, preferably with water (boiling, soups, stews and steaming) to bring an expansive quality to the foods.
7. **Thin, Small** Use building and invigorating foods. Steamed grains and congee help build Blood and Fluids, but on their own don't provide movement. Use ginger and chives to add movement. Green vegetables build Blood and provide directionality. Bean soup: lentil, mung or adzuki (large beans are likely to cause stagnation). Comfort foods are important if the pulse is thin. If the patient's comfort food is chicken soup or meat, care must be taken that Heat doesn't build up and deplete Blood.
8. **Choppy** Use congee with warming spices. Cooked apple with cinnamon and clove.

9. **Rough** Build Blood to clear internal Wind, perhaps with blueberries, red grapes.

10. **Narrow, Fine** Nourish whichever mediumship is deficient, indicated by the level at which the narrowness was found.

11. **Big, Wide** Leave as it is.

12. **Short** Build the mediumship indicated. Eventually, open with leafy vegetables and spices.

13. **Long** Strengthen the Spleen/Pancreas by reducing Damp and adding foods with a Spleen affinity. (See above, Slippery or Long pulses.)

14. **Slippery** First reduce the foods that most often create Dampness: sugar, dairy, and glutinous grains. Increase foods that strengthen the Spleen/Pancreas such as sweet potato, squash, and congee-type porridges. Ice, hot peppers, or alcohol can also be dietary factors contributing to the slippery pulse. After reducing or eliminating these, foods to drain Dampness will be more effective: mushrooms, small beans, sprouts. Sleep, stress, worry, and timing of meals can also be key factors in weakening digestion manifesting as a slippery pulse.

15. **Beady** Break up hardnesses with foods classified as salty, including seaweeds.

16. **Not Rested** Any foods that boost Kidney energetics will help: nuts, shellfish, seaweed, mushrooms. Also use adzuki beans to foster communication between Heart and Kidneys.

17. **Empty** Build Qi and mediumship with good diet, carefully monitored to insure good digestion and assimilation of that diet.

18. **Faint, Frail** Showing as it does in the guan position, the pulse texture faint or frail indicates Blood and Qi deficiency. If in the right guan position, nourish Blood with grains (select appropriate to digestion strength), green leafy vegetables, beets, berries and beef or bison, favoring wet preparations such as congee, soups, stews. (These can include stewed berries or other fruits, to maximize absorption and avoid cooling the digestive tract). If faint or frail in the left guan, focus on strengthening capacity to bank and manage Blood, using tart berries (including goji, blueberries, raspberries, etc.), ascending vegetables (asparagus), citrus peel, and vinegar (brined foods).

19. **Scattered** Consolidate Qi with roasted beets, carrots, parsnips, brussels sprouts, etc., fermented foods, nuts, seeds.

20. **Leathery, Taut** Use sour foods to restrain leakages: pickles, vinegar, fermented foods. Fine-tune to the level of leakage by mixing sour foods with signature foods, e.g., sunflower seeds for Middle Jiao and Blood (roasted to increase Yang/strength) with lemon juice.

21. **Firm** Use sour to secure Jing-Essence: sorrel, seeds with vinegar, lambs lettuce, chicory, endive, radicchio with lemon juice or vinegar.

22. **Hidden** First, make clinical decision whether to support latency or help bring out

and rid a pathogenic factor. To support latency, consolidate Qi and mediumship with soups, stews, congee, bone broths, compact vegetables, and cooling foods such as bitter greens and sprouts (still cooked, though lightly). The capacity for latency can be increased by carefully cooling the Zang Fu—slowing damage due to Heat—using grains, sprouts, bitter greens, and perhaps juices. Include spices like fresh ginger and turmeric to protect digestion from cooling foods.

If the decision is to rid the pathogen, use diet to support a Divergent strategy (Superficial-Deep-Superficial) by carefully stimulating Wei Qi and Yuan Qi simultaneously, while providing movement and elimination. Use of sea vegetables, spices, seeds, mushrooms, nuts, sprouts and beans is important, along with bitter greens to help clear fire toxins as they emerge. Identify the specific level to be cleared and apply signature foods. Small amounts of foods such as dairy that tend to stimulate Wei Qi can be useful for some. Monitor pulses carefully. This requires careful knowledge of food energetics and a clear assessment of the strength of the patient. If not sure, simply build mediumship with congee, grains and broths while protecting against food stagnation with vegetables, sprouts and spices.

Another approach, perhaps the simplest and most important, is not to engage in therapy directly but to treat counterflow Qi if it arises (using fresh ginger and root vegetable soups). Food stagnation and constipation must be treated if they arise; elimination must be open when clearing pathogenic factors.

23. **Moving, Vibrating** Use foods that resonate with Jing-Essence: mollusks, sea vegetables, seeds, nuts, eggs, mushrooms. Combine leafy greens with sesame seeds or walnuts.

24. **Normal** Celebrate.

25. **Superficial** Assist Wei Qi with cinnamon, mint and scallion while building fluids with congee.

26. **Floating, Flooding, Surging** If there is excess Wei Qi activity, assist with cinnamon, mint and scallion while building fluids with congee. If Yang Qi is rising to escape, help anchor with nuts, root vegetables, short grains, shellfish, fish, and bone broth.

27. **Hollow, Scallion** Tightness at the superficial and deep levels with a hollow (at least not tight) feeling in the middle indicates the need to either nourish Blood or astringe Blood in cases of leakage. Build Blood with grains, leafy vegetables, beets, berries and meat (especially beef or bison). To astringe or contain leakage, use short grain or sticky rice (to hold in) or wheat (if well tolerated), along with tart berries and stalk vegetables that strengthen Yang Qi.

28. **Soft** A soft pulse lacks integrity and signifies the need for consolidation. Strengthen

the Spleen/Pancreas to support acupuncture or herbal strategy. Buckwheat is useful as a temporary staple grain to support the integrity of the Blood vessels themselves if they are also involved.

29. **Urgent** To clear gu and entities, clear Phlegm and Dampness by abstaining from sugar, dairy, sticky grains while adding bitter greens and small beans. Nourish the Heart with adzuki beans, pistachios, etc.

30. **Hasty** Use clams, abalone, seed spices and black sesame seeds to clear Heat in the Yuan level.

31. **Knotted** Use seed spices (cumin, caraway, cardamom, fennel seed, etc.) to warm the Yuan level.

32. **Intermittent** Calm Shen with pistachio and lotus seed, connect Heart and Kidney with adzuki beans and black sesame seeds,while restoring enthusiasm with warming digestive spices and vegetables with an ascending vector.

FURTHER CONSIDERATIONS

DIRECTIONALITY

Diet is very important for the directionality of internal energy.

1. If the ascending vector of the Spleen is weak or absent, include ascending vegetables: asparagus, the stems of vegetables (broccoli stems or Chinese broccoli, chard stems, kohlrabi, etc.), sweet potato to strengthen the Spleen, and uplifting kitchen herbs such as rosemary.

2. If the Stomach is not descending or accepting food well: root vegetables, leafy green vegetables such as collard, chard, kale (they spread, but are also cool so support descension). Also, carrots, beets, daikon, burdock. Rice, steamed or as congee, harmonizes the Stomach and Spleen/pancreas, including Spleen ascension and Stomach descension.

3. If the Lungs are not dispersing/effusing sufficiently: scallions, radishes, mustard greens, arugula, and kitchen herbs including dill, oregano, basil, mustard seed.

4. If the Lungs are not descending: root vegetables such as daikon, parsnip, carrot. Seeds such as sesame seeds anchor Lung Qi. Apples and pears aid descension if eaten raw (check the status of the Spleen). Fiber connects with the Large Intestine, Lung's Yang pair.

5. If the Liver is ascending too much: drain Liver Fire with bitter vegetables (also useful to open the Stomach) including artichoke, olives, watercress, endive, dandelion greens, brussels sprouts. Mung Bean sprouts also drain Liver and Gallbladder Heat. Avoid foods that stagnate or constrain the Liver. If there is too little Liver ascension, add wine to the cooking, increase asparagus, etc.

6. If the Triple Heater is floating: drain Fire Toxins with bitter and root vegetables such as burdock, dandelion, kale, Chinese broccoli, bitter melon, broccoli rabe, etc. Avoid nightshades, garlic, other foods that Heat the Blood.

7. If the Heart is not dispersing well: open with red kale, mustard greens, warming spices such as cumin seeds, adzuki beans. Nourish the Heart with adzukis, lotus seeds, etc.

8. If the Liver is not nourishing the Kidneys (Liver descending), use beans (as they work with Blood and as the link between the Yuan and Ying levels), seaweed, rice, greens, sesame seeds, chestnuts or walnuts.

9. If the Heart is not communicating with the Kidneys, use lotus seeds, adzuki beans, radicchio, in careful combination such as bitter greens with walnuts that have been quick-fried with honey (to clear the Heart but also to enliven Qi and rouse enthusiasm). In all cases, the cooking method and food combination is important.

10. Blockage between pulses: diaphragm may be most common, use bitter greens such as dandelion, chicory, arugula, endive, broccoli rabe. Above chest: spinach unbinds the chest. Below the diaphragm would include premenstrual stress, or difficulty beginning menstruation: all these greens are appropriate.

11. Refusal: first consider blockages, then diagnose the source of the refusal with keen attention to emotional complexities. Use Heart foods already mentioned, or invigorate Blood (a Luo dietary strategy) with goji berries, warming spices, seed spices, scallion, leek or chive. If grief is present, use dill, almonds, pine nuts.

12. If a healing crisis: explore comfort foods that will not impede the healing strategy. Dairy, sugar, gluten and certain nuts will slow the healing crisis, so look for comfort foods that are less sticky, if possible. Use Kidney affinity foods to help a person restore the sense of who they are and that life is good. Consider walnuts, chestnuts, black rice, black sesame seeds, and something to provide movement once grounding is improved, such as scallions, chives, and cumin to foster self-expression.

HOW TO INTEGRATE DIET FOR TREATMENTS OF SINEW, LUO, DIVERGENT AND EIGHT EXTRAORDINARY CHANNELS (EXCEPTIONALLY BRIEF INTRODUCTION):

1. To support Sinew Channel treatments, use warming/spreading/invigorating spices to direct pathogenic factors out (cinnamon, nutmeg, clove, scallion, etc.) Fluids may need support through congee.

2. To support Luo Channel treatments, invigorate blood with chives, blueberries paired with mint or dill, blood oranges with pistachio nuts dusted with cumin. Full diagnosis is necessary, but this may help point a way.

3. To support Divergent Channel treatments, first decide if food should help clear a

deep pathogenic factor or help support its latency. The difference is achieved through using foods with affinities for Yuan Level (nuts, beans, seafood, eggs) and Wei Level (spices, fruit, some nuts and seeds, eggs) then combining them in careful balance with very clear cooking and eating intention. To support latency (Deep-Superficial-Deep), use walnuts cooked with honey, bone broths, or dairy such as potato/clam/milk chowder (without black pepper). Use consolidating foods and cooking method. To bring out for clearing (Superficial-Deep-Superficial) use almonds or pine nuts warmed with oil and spices (cinnamon, cardamom, cumin) to open the Lungs and push the pathogenic factor out. Use eggs with what seems like too much chive, rosemary, oregano and other warming spices. Care must be taken with every food at these times; for example, habit foods such as chocolate or peanuts can ruin Divergent treatments if latency support is the strategy, while dairy or sugar could ruin the treatment if clearing is the strategy. An important role for diet in any clearing strategy is to insure that elimination is not stagnated (e.g., food stagnation, constipation, water retention or urinary issues). Before beginning a clearing strategy, assess elimination and prepare the body through appropriate clearing strategies.

4. To support Eight Extra treatments, support Yuan Level and provide help consolidating (with beans, certain nuts, preserved foods, seaweeds, roasted vegetables or meats). Use or avoid spices (especially seed spices) and ascending or wide-leaf vegetables in a strategy to invigorate or not, as appropriate. To support the hormonal level, be sure to include plenty of good quality fats and oils: olive oil, nut oils, seed oils or butter.

INDIVIDUAL PATIENT ASSESSMENT: INTEGRATION OF PULSES AND DIET

At its best, all medicine is individual medicine. The unique individuality of the patient is beyond any limits or preconceptions. This is the essence of the clinical encounter.

Dietary advice must be individual. Dietary counsel depends upon good diagnosis and knowledge of food energetics, not on theories of good diets or "what is good for you." With a patient, the question is "Let's see how your diet is working for you, in your pulses and through seeing your tongue." Chinese Medicine never recommends a standardized "diet" in any way.

When looking through the lens of diet, assess the following through pulse diagnosis:
1. Signs of Cold, Heat (inflammation) or both.
2. How are Grains doing for the individual? (Examine the effect of grains, pasta, bread, breakfast cereals or baked goods, snacks, etc.) Look for slippery pulses, Spleen Yang ascension issues, etc.
3. What is the status of Fluids? Sufficient hydration, signs of Dampness? Where is Dampness or Phlegm coming from? Is it resulting from not handling the intake of

carbs, sugar, dairy, alcohol? Are there sleep issues impacting Kidney Yang and its role in supporting the Spleen/Pancreas?

4. Is digestion working well? Are the Stomach and Spleen ascending Pure Yang and Fluids to the Upper Jiao?

5. Is there sufficient Blood?

6. Is the Liver Constrained?

7. Is there Wind?

8. Is there stagnation in the Lower Jiao? If so, food and elimination, blood, hormonal or a combination?

9. How does the complaint and associated signs & symptoms relate to the impact you think the individual's diet might have on them?

10. What is the emotional state of the patient and how does it weave in with digestion and the complaint?

Then, discuss recommendations regarding:

1. Grains

2. Vegetables

3. Animal Foods

4. Dairy

5. Spices

6. Things that may cause problems: Sugar, Hot Spices, Alcohol, Coffee, Chocolate, Tea, or anything that is a dietary compulsion. Help patient look at what they reach for everyday—that's the food & drink that may be holding them in place.

7. Cooking Methods (should match therapeutic strategy)

8. Constructing dishes, meals and how to implement what is recommended into a successful dietary plan.

CHAPTER 9

CASES

My patient has floating and tight pulses in all three positions on the right wrist but they are not moving pulses. The Spleen pulse is rapid at the moderate and superficial levels. There is a lot of Qi moving not just from Spleen to Lung but back to the Spleen from the Lung. The Lung pulse is rapid on the moderate level and full on the deep level. At the superficial level, however, it is discernibly slower. The moderate level of the Heart pulse is soft; it gives way when I press beyond nine beans. The Liver pulse is slippery. The left Kidney pulse is floating and tight. What might be happening in this scenario?

R   L

_____   _____
_____ rapid _____ LU   HT _____
_____ full _____   _____

____ floating, tight, rapid ____   _____
_____ rapid _____ SP   LR _____ slippery _____
_____   _____

_____   _____
_____ floating, tight _____   _____ floating, tight _____
_____ KI Yang   KI Yin _____
_____   _____

The back and forth between the Spleen and Lungs means that the guan position is trying to pass pathology up and out, but the Lungs keep sending it back. Perhaps they don't want to express it. The pathological factor is building up in the Lungs and we know that it is not being expressed because the superficial level of the Lung pulse is not also rapid. In fact, because the superficial Lung pulse is slower, the factor is trapped. Whenever the guan position has a rapid or floating quality, the cun position must be floating in order to vent that pathology. This is likely an emotional situation. The patient is unable to express the emotion and the build up of that Qi is causing Heat to build up in the Upper Jiao. The danger here is that the Heat can become trapped in the breast. You could release ST-19 and SI-1 to get the Heat to vent from the breast.

While the right guan shows its urgent quest to release pathology from the guan, on the left side the Heart pulse is soft; it's showing that it wants to maintain latency. This means the latency the Heart displays is of the emotions; the Heart does not want to express the emotions. You might bleed the Luo Channels to get the emotions to vent. The Liver deals with courage. Perhaps she is not able to muster the fortitude to deal with the repression. The tension in the Sinews showing in all three positions may be there to block the expression of Yuan-Source Qi to the Bladder Shu points. Your patient might consider that life is painful.

CASE 2

My new patient presents with the following pulses. The cun positions on both wrists are very full at the moderate level. The guan positions are each floating and tight at the Wei level. When I check to see if the Spleen is ascending to the Lungs, instead of the vector becoming evident, the area between the guan and cun positions swells into a mound and the pulse becomes rapid in the guan position. The right chi position is tight at the moderate level. On the left, the Heart and Kidneys are not communicating. The Liver is empty and does not communicate to the Heart or the Kidneys. The Spleen is rough at the moderate level. After I press to 15 beans, the pulse is moving and long in the left chi position. What might be happening here?

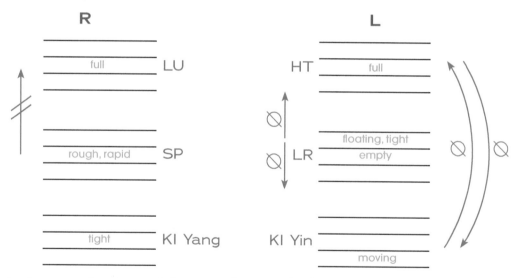

The bulge between the guan and the cun indicates a diaphragmatic blockage. As you check the vector between the Spleen and the Lungs, the Spleen shows its willingness to ascend to the Lungs but the diaphragm is not letting it through. It tries to move, but simply becomes rapid because it cannot move. Just as Qi is unable to go upward across the diaphragm, so too is it unable to descend past the diaphragm. Qi is therefore trapped in the Upper Jiao, causing both cun pulses to be full, or congested. This Inter-Jiao blockage is also preventing communication between the Heart and Kidneys. The Pericardium is also tightening, and that too will prevent communication between the Heart and Kidneys. It may be having an impact on its Jue Yin pair, the Liver and contributing to the tightness at the diaphragm. The rough Spleen suggests there is too much thinking, churning of the mind and the patient feels very unsettled. All this mental activity has depleted the Blood and there is Wind resulting. This patient is likely to experience anxiety, palpitations, an unpleasant fullness in the chest. They might be worrying about the past and unable to be in present time since there is a Yin Wei Mai pulse present (long, moving pulse in the chi position). Communicate the Heart and Kidney, unblock the diaphragm (LR-14 or BL-17 will do this) and nourish all Blood perhaps with the entire trajectory of Yin Wei Mai.

CASE 3

My patient has cancer and prominent ascites which is very painful for him. He is receiving chemotherapy. The Spleen pulse at the superficial level is floating and slightly tight. At the moderate level, it's very tight and thin. (His lips are dry, by the way.) At the deep level, it's also tight and slightly thin. His Lung pulse is deep and scattered and does not and will not float. It hits my finger at several locations. The Kidney pulses are both weak. The right Kidney pulse is floating and very rapid. The Heart pulse is floating and slightly tight at the superficial level. The Liver pulse is slippery on the moderate level and rapid on the deep level. What might be the big picture here?

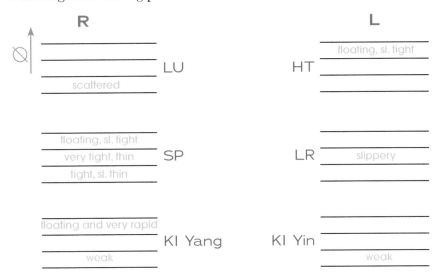

The right cun shows the Lungs have not been releasing pathology. The scattered pulse at the deep level means Lung Qi cannot descend. The Kidney pulses are weak on both sides, so the Kidneys don't have the capacity to grasp Lung Qi anyway. This patient is very tired. There are floating and tight pulses in the guan and cun positions, so there is significant shoulder tension. The rapidity in these pulses shows that the body is creating Heat to try to move the Sinews in the shoulder region and possibly other regions. These need to be released. The moderate level of the right guan is tight and thin, indicating deficiency of Fluids and an attempt to conserve what Fluids are available. The ascites is manifesting this. Don't attempt to drain that fluid, but hydrate the patient so that the ascites has no reason to be there. Water with lemon in it will help the body astringe Fluids so that the pathological fluids can be released. ST-24 needled now will help him separate the pure from the turbid and assist in timely release. If the right guan is tight and thin, it might not be making Blood sufficiently, or it might not be able to manage Blood. There may be leakage of blood, or bruising. The floating, rapid, right chi pulse indicates metastasis. The treatment here could be Triple Heater Divergent Channel deep-superficial-deep to secure latency while you restore mediumship and Qi.

CASE 4

On the right wrist, my elderly patient has full pulses at the moderate and deep levels of the cun position. It does not float. The guan is floating, tight and rapid at the moderate level and rapid at the deep level. The right chi is weak. There is a very full and long pulse on the deep level joining the cun and guan positions. On the left wrist, the left cun is unremarkable. The left guan is tight and floating on the superficial level and full and tight on the moderate level. On the deep level, the guan is tight and slightly full. The left chi pulses are found on the deep level where they should be, but are weak. When I press down on the Lung pulse, the guan becomes stronger. The Kidneys do not grasp Lung Qi.

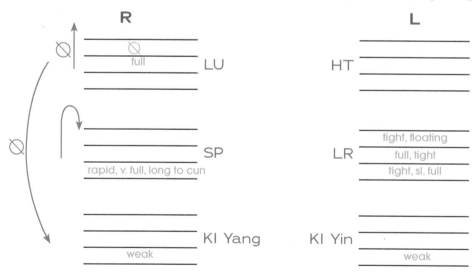

As we become older, the pulses tend to become fuller. Geriatrics is very similar to pediatrics, but the elderly have true deficiencies, while children have insufficiencies; they haven't developed the resources in the first place. In geriatrics, it's imperative that postnatal Qi is able to nourish prenatal Qi. First, descend the Lungs to the Kidneys so that Da Qi can reach the Kidneys. Encourage the use of root vegetables in the diet. The Lungs are full but not floating; there is Qi building up. At the same time, the left guan is floating, full and tight; pathology is potentially moving to the brain. Stroke is a possibility. There may be scalp tension. Move the Large Intestine to help this Qi move down. Taro root, or oatmeal with almonds move stagnation in the bowels. The deep level of the left guan was full and tight, so there's a lot of activity in the Middle Jiao. There could be rebellious Qi in the

Middle Jiao, or excessive thinking. Bleed SP-4, the Luo point before you continue with your treatment.

CASE 5: ONLY THE PULSES WILL TELL

For many years I'd been seeing a patient who presents with depression. Usually I find her Lung pulse only on the deep level. After treatment, it disperses and she is free of depression for about 90 days. Today she told me that she had spent a week sleeping about 18 hours a day, sleep that was divided into groups of several hours separated by periods of waking rest. She said she needed help with lethargy. On this particular day, the pulses were unlike any of her previous presentations. I found nothing in any position in the moderate or superficial levels and very little in the deep level. I press down to 15 beans to see whether she was inviting a treatment at the Eight Extra level and found a very strong Chong Mai pulse. I suggested that her pulse invited the movement of Kidney Yang to the Spleen and that the invitation was occurring at a very deep level, a level at which the cycles of life were addressed. She replied that she was about to turn 50 and it felt as though a major transition was about to occur. I asked whether she might need help with that transition and she readily agreed.

Needling into SP-4, I noticed that the point seemed to grasp the needle and pull it in and up. She reported that she felt an immediate sense of calm. I read the pulses again and found that for the first time since I had known her, all the pulses were fully communicating with each other, and each pulse was at its theoretically correct depth. I proceeded to the next point on the first trajectory, CV-2. The point refused the needle, walling itself off as though in a protective stance. Exactly the same thing happened at KI-11. Chong Mai was resisting treatment because SP-4 had brought the channel into alignment and there was no need to go any further with that channel. There had to be another message here. One point cannot constitute a treatment since treatment is about creating a relationship between points. I asked the patient if she had any idea what the nature of her transition into the next chapter might be. She'd had vivid images of her instant death in a car accident on the highway and had made a will the previous week. She was certain the next chapter was going involve the completion of this life.

I told her that her pulses were in perfect alignment, like a musical instrument and that there was no hint of depression in them. (The Lungs were strong and fully dispersing.) She agreed that there had been an enormous shift on the table but wanted an explanation for the lethargy that had been so debilitating of late. As we are preparing to end a life, we rehearse for the transition by sleeping more and more. But significant periods of somnolence can also precede new chapters in the continuation of this lifetime. Images of death can, of course, be symbolic of the end of a chapter, the end of a mindset, the 'death' of a way of being. I told her that she might be preparing for the next chapter by amassing the resources needed to move into the next cycle of ten years. She agreed and asked for help stabilizing so that she could embrace her path. I took the pulses again in order to work out where I was being invited. She showed a clear Yang Wei Mai pulse. I needled it with the intention of helping her view the future with positive expectation. As she was leaving, she very casually gave me a hug (unusual), looked me in the eye and said "Goodbye". Before the end of the week she was offered an interesting job in another country.

CASE 6: THE PULSE RULES

Occasionally I have trouble finding any pulse at all. Nothing in the Wei level, nothing in the Ying level, nothing in the Yuan level. Usually, with further palpation, looking for Hidden or Moving pulses yields a pulse but sometimes it doesn't. Since it is Yang that causes the pulse to arise, one must investigate why Yang is not evident in the pulses. Recently this happened during the examination of a patient of happy disposition who is an athlete, a successful businesswoman, cooks all her own food and had just returned from a vacation in the tropics with her extended family. As I was taking the pulses, I asked how her trip was. She said she had enjoyed a perfect time in the sun, relaxing and being with the family. As she spoke this sentence, the Liver pulse suddenly appeared, tight and rapid in the moderate level. I reported this to her and asked whether anything frustrating happened on the trip. After quite a while she told me that her son hid an illicit substance in her luggage before the return journey. She found it the previous evening while unpacking, confronted him, and was bereft with what she felt was betrayal. Very deep disappointment can cause the withdrawal of the pulses, as though the Heart is frozen. To return the pulses to their expressive height, I needled and vibrated The Guest House, KI-9, a point that enables the patient to be in present time.

CASE 7: THE PULSE IS OPTIMISTIC

An exhausted woman arrived at my office having just been released from a day in the hospital. She had been suffering severe headaches and reported that her blood pressure was 200/120. Tests in the ER showed she had IgA nephropathy, was seriously anemic, and to her great surprise, pregnant. Her kidneys were functioning at 25% capacity. She would not be a candidate for a kidney transplant "until" her kidney function declined to 10%. Her doctors estimated that to be about two years away. They said the pregnancy would have to be terminated because the risk of a stroke was high, the kidneys would likely fail, and she would have a miscarriage anyway. When she arrived I listened to her account and went to the pulses, keeping my mind clear and open to all possibilities. There was wonderful news: the Spleen was ascending strongly. Or was it? Could I be feeling the Stomach ascending or Yang escaping, rising up, causing the hypertension? Could it be that the pregnancy was in fact a time bomb, that both mother and child were at risk? I checked to see whether the Stomach was descending; if the strength of the Stomach's descending vector matched the strength of the Spleen's ascending vector, I could deduce that I was feeling the Spleen valiantly holding the pregnancy up. The Stomach was indeed descending, and strongly. The Kidney pulses, however, were extremely rapid. I could not slow them with my intention during palpation of the pulses. The pathology was contained in the kidney organ itself.

Indeed, the patient had a history of urinary tract infections that tended to move up into the kidneys. I searched the Divergent pulses. Sure enough, the Kidney Divergent pulse was present. I decided to treat that channel, to bring the Kidney pathology into latency. In one week, both the protein level in the urine and the creatinine halved. Dialysis was not needed at any point. Weekly treatment of that channel was maintained. At week 27, the patient was told she would certainly develop pre-eclampsia, that there was no chance of any other outcome. Her doctor promised his entire staff and interns breakfast in the diner across the road if the patient made it to 36 weeks; he could not explain how a patient with kidney failure could proceed through pregnancy without complication. The treatments were holding the pathology away from the kidneys. Breakfast was served at 36 weeks! At 37 weeks she did develop pre-eclampsia and was given a C-section. Baby was perfect. Treatment continued as needed for several years until the patient moved to Europe with her husband and healthy child.

CASE 8: KEEP IT SIMPLE

Scenario: Your patient arrives 38 minutes late for his one hour session. You want to quickly find a valid diagnosis that would enable you to perform a meaningful treatment. First look for superficial tight pulses. If you find any, ask about pain, stiffness or difficulty making particular movements. Release the appropriate Jing Well points. If there are no superficial tight pulses, check that the cun pulses are dispersing, coming up into the Wei level. If they are not, put your focus there. If you find rapid pulses in the guan position and the cun is not floating, the body is unable to express Heat and the Heat may become trapped. If the cun is floating and the guan is not showing a rapid pulse, proceed to the Spleen position. Treat any pathological qualities you find there. Tonifying the Spleen will benefit every aspect of health and doesn't take long!

CASE 9: THE WAY IS LIGHTED

Sometimes treatment choices are unequivocally present in the pulses. A 13-year-old boy presented with anxiety. His Lung pulse was not detectable, the Spleen was deep and rapid and the right Kidney pulse was rapid tight and at the moderate level. Even before I took the left pulses, it was clear that something had alarmed him but that he felt powerless to act; he had withdrawn (Lung pulse was retracted) but the panic was overwhelming (the Kidney pulse was rapid and tight). The left pulses were extraordinarily clear; there were no pulses in the Ying and Wei levels but the left wrist showed a strong moving pulse in the cun position. The pulse there was moving steadily, laterally from side to side, one beat close to the tendon and then the following beat away from the tendon, the next close to the tendon again, and the next, away. This is the Yang Qiao Mai pulse. Given the right wrist pulses, I asked him whether he had received some bad news or whether he had experienced something unsettling. He said that the previous day he had visited an orthodontist who told him that his jaw was too small (underdeveloped) and that he must have four teeth extracted soon, otherwise his mouth would become overcrowded, preventing chewing. I suggested that his natural rate of growth might not match the schedule of most teenagers, that he might be a late bloomer, and that the orthodontist might be persuaded to wait and see. These ideas were not welcomed; the appointment to remove four teeth had been made as it was considered a matter of urgency. I negotiated a 90 day delay. The way forward was illuminated by the Yang Qiao Mai pulse in the left wrist and I wanted to follow its call to address that marvelous channel that aligns the structure. After three months, the boy returned to his astonished orthodontist who measured the jaw and found it the perfect size, ample and ready to welcome his burgeoning teeth.

CASE 10: THE LEVELS TELL A STORY

A 19-year-old woman presented with regular minor strokes, causing what appeared to be permanent, partial paralysis of her right arm, shoulder and leg. Lupus had been diagnosed at age 14, lupus nephritis at age 17, and the current Western diagnosis was central nervous system lupus vasculitis. Every few weeks she would have strokes of varying severity, some requiring hospitalization. The strokes were precipitated by some kind of reaching or stretching such as reaching for toilet paper, a towel, a can of beans on a shelf. One month prior to her acupuncture visit she had had a major stroke resulting in permanent partial paralysis of the right side. She was covered in a fine rash all over her torso and arms. I asked her what was going on when she was 14. She said that her parents fought about their failing business for years and that at age 12 she was sent to boarding school where she was desperately unhappy, was bullied, and suffered from chronic insomnia. Two years in, she began having strokes.

The Spleen pulse appeared slightly rapid and tight on the moderate level, but when pressed to the deep level, it increased to 17 beats per breath. There was Heat trapped in the Spleen. The vector between the Spleen and Lungs was absent. Qi, and therefore the Heat was not able to vent from the Middle to the Upper Jiao. Or was it? The Lung pulse was tight and rapid also, but was not floating. There was Heat trapped in the Lungs also; the deep level was at about 14 beats per breath. So perhaps some of the Heat had been transferred to the Upper Jiao. The patient was a living pressure cooker. The pulses were very thin. The Heat had consumed Blood and Fluids. Wind had entered the channels, and strokes were the result of the intermittent attempts the body made to evacuate the Wind and the Heat. I told the patient that she had so much Heat, she had the pulses of someone who ate garlic and onions every day. She immediately said "I do!". Her mother cooked lovingly, being sure to add lots of garlic, believing it to be beneficial.

The Kidney pulse on the right side was leathery and floating at the same time. Yang Qi was escaping. On the left side, all three positions were superficial and rapid, sitting at one bean of pressure. On further palpation, the Liver was not ascending to the Heart. The failure of the Middle Jiao to ascend to the Upper Jiao on both wrists indicated a possible diaphragmatic blockage. It would be unwise to release that before Heat was released directly from the Middle Jiao because the Heat could then spontaneously rise to the Upper Jiao and overwhelm it. I elected to bleed ST-40 to release the Heat, and then released the diaphragm at BL-17 and LR-14. The rash disappeared within a few days. Over the next few weeks we worked first on nourishing Yin and Blood and then on clearing Wind while the patient adopted a spice-free, deeply hydrating wet diet featuring mild soups and stews. The patient has not experienced strokes in the years since the treatments.

CASE 11: LET THE PULSES TALK

One morning a patient arrived in great pain, bent over, unable to straighten his back. The pain was one-sided, chronic and intermittent. The pulses were wiry at the moderate level of the Liver position and tight at the deep level of the left and right Kidney pulses. Pressure applied to the Liver position at the deep level caused the Kidney pulse to tighten even more. It appeared the tension was originating in the Liver. I asked the patient whether he was angry. He denied it as I continued to palpate the pulses, inviting the Liver to give up its tension. After a couple of minutes, he said angrily, "Well, anyone would be angry trying to get into Manhattan at 9am on a Friday!" The Liver began to release as the frustration was being expressed outwardly. I invited him to lie on the table but didn't specify whether he should be face down or face up. (The table was set up for both.) He got up from the sofa, straightened his back effortlessly without realizing it, and lay down on the table, face up. The manipulation of the pulses had released most of the pathology. Then, in placing himself on the table face-up, the patient was acting in alignment with his pulses; the treatment needed to be focussed on the Middle Jiao, not the back. The treatment to calm and free the Middle Jiao completed the healing that began with the taking of the pulses.

CASE 12: PULSES AND PLANNING

Acupuncture treatments cannot be planned. Each treatment must correspond with the pulse findings of that day. Each day, the pulses are unique. Careful pulse taking ensures awareness of the changes a patient is undergoing during treatment, indicates what resources you have to work with that day, and enables you to switch gears to follow and guide their individual healing trajectory with certainty.

A woman presented with acute rheumatoid arthritis. The condition arose the day after a round of injections that were part of the IVF procedure. The pulses were weak and rapid in the moderate level of the Liver pulse. The Lungs, Kidneys and Spleen were weak and difficult to find, and she was in a tremendous amount of pain. The joints were red, swollen and so painful she was unable to use them. She was exhausted and tremendously dispirited. One option would be to release heat and tonify Qi, but on further palpation, there was a Hidden, Moving pulse in the left guan position. I first released some of the Heat by bleeding some Luo points, then needled the Liver and Gallbladder Divergent Channel deep-superficial-deep, to invite the condition into latency while her resources were rebuilt. Each week the pulses showed steady improvement and surprising changes. Every class of channel presented in the pulse over the first six weeks. Ultimately, the pulses became superficial and Heat began to express as capillaries all over her legs and arms. Adhering to the pulse findings that were unique each week resulted in no two treatments being the same. The pulses were shining the light, guiding the way through the patient's individual maze of illness. The rheumatoid arthritis was almost completely cleared within three months. The only vestiges of the disease were ganglion cysts that emerged in the hands toward the end. The patient was pregnant in the fourth month after treatment commenced. The cysts dissolved in the second trimester. Labor lasted two hours and baby was perfect.

CHAPTER 10

PULSES IN CHILDREN

Diagnosis in children differs from that of adults in that the radial artery is seldom examined. Instead, a variety of techniques can be used. The standard pulses at the radial artery yield clear readings in children three years of age and over. Sometimes the pulses become readable when the child begins walking. Pulse rates should always be compared with respiration to contextualize the apparent rapidity of pulses in the very young, as they naturally have higher pulse rates than adults. This is not an indicator of Heat. Rather, it's a mark of the Heart's effort to become comfortable with the environment, the new life and its setting. Tremendous amounts of Yang are coming to the surface to enable the quest to understand the world. Yang emerges as curiosity abounds; the child's nature is finding ground, becoming stabilized. This exuberance of Yang is normal. Only after puberty does the pulse rate near the adult rate. Pulse rates change at the time of menses as the accompanying comparatively Yin state brings them down.

Prior to the age of three, diagnosis has several components including examination of the index finger, the area between the eyes, the area superior to that—sometimes called the third eye—the carotid artery and the ears.

DIAGNOSIS AT THE INDEX FINGER

The principal site of diagnosis in children under three years is the index finger, which is rubbed gently to reveal the color of the veins in the fingers. Interestingly, the concept of diagnosing by looking at the complexion evolved from pediatric diagnosis. Analysis of the finger is felt to be superior to analysis of the complexion because a child's complexion can change quickly and unpredictably.

The finger is divided into segments in alignment with the Jiaos: the cun, guan, and chi. The three joints of the finger are known as: the Wind Gate, the Qi Gate and Life Gate.

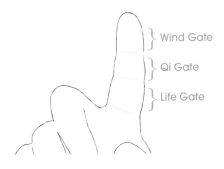

Wind Gate

Qi Gate

Life Gate

The index finger is rubbed along the edge of its anterior surface to stimulate the surfacing of a vein:

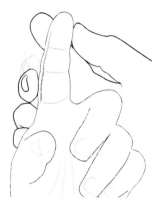

Engorged or strongly colored veins indicate imbalances in the three Jiaos. As in the pulses of the wrist, the left finger is Yin and maps Kidney Yin, Liver and Heart. The right finger is Yang and maps Kidney Yang, the digestive tract and the Lungs. Often the finger needs to be pulled back slightly to stretch the vein a little to make it more visible.

- The state of the vein in the Life Gate of the index finger reveals the state of Lower Jiao and of Yuan Qi.
- The state of the vein in the Qi Gate of the index finger reveals the state of the Middle Jiao and of Ying Qi.
- The state of the veins in the Wind Gate of the index finger reveals the state of the region superior to the diaphragm including the head and any Wind activity or propensity for Wind.
- A blue vein indicates stagnation, Yang deficiency, Cold or a combination of the above. If the vein is deep at the same time, Yang deficiency or Cold are likely. If the vein does not look deep in the finger but is dark in color, the apparent stagnation is likely a result of Cold.
- Dark veins on the finger indicate stagnation.
- A bright red vein indicates Heat.
- A blue vein in the top joint indicates the presence of Wind. In children, this may affect the psyche, the Hun and the dissemination of Yuan Qi. Note that often what we might consider Liver signs are simply signs of the failure of the Lungs to control Qi.
- A blue vein in the Qi Gate indicates Cold in the digestive tract. There could be abdominal pain or upset, food sensitivity, intolerance to formula, sometimes even intolerance to the mother's breast milk (usually caused by the mother's diet).
- An engorged reddish or bluish vein at Life Gate on the index finger indicates

Heat or stagnation in the Yuan level. This is common, since Yang Qi is not yet fully articulated in the very young.

- By about 18 months of age, the vein usually becomes bluish due to vaccinations.

Luo points are bled to release Heat, Cold or to move stagnation.

The findings in the index fingers are combined with the findings at Ming Tang, that is, the area between the eyes also known as The Hall of Brightness, described on page 188.

CAROTID ARTERY DIAGNOSIS IN CHILDREN

The pulses can be read at ST-9 until the age of three, or until the child begins teething and assimilating solid food, today commonly earlier than three years of age. The notion that children have big pulses comes from the observation that the pulse at ST-9 becomes more pronounced under the influence of pathology. A common challenge to the immune system is the early introduction of unfamiliar milk. The body can read this as a pathological invasion if introduced too early.

If the pulse at the carotid artery is twice as big as the radial artery, the condition is said to be in Shao Yang. If it is three times as big as the radial artery, it is said to be in Tai Yang. If four times as big the condition is in Yang Ming and is potentially serious.

Palpation of the carotid artery was common, classically. The left carotid pulse at ST-9 is referred to as Ren Ying, the Welcoming of Humanity. Right ST-9 is known as the Mouth of Qi. ST-9 reflects movements of Qi. ST-9 on the left side gives the status of the Stomach while the right ST-9 gives the status of the intestines and the Spleen. Together they reflect how well the Stomach and Spleen or the Stomach and intestines are harmonized.

The pulse at ST-9 is compared to the pulse at LU-9. If the pulse at ST-9 has greater strength or is more rapid than LU-9 there is rebellious Qi. The child should be given smaller meals several times a day. Large meals would stagnate Qi, creating accumulations and negatively impacting growth. If the right ST-9 has more strength than LU-9, there is Dampness in the intestines.[1] The child should not be given any sugar as this will lead to early dental problems. They should be given more water to irrigate the intestines. Long-term imbalances of the Stomach and Spleen or intestines causes Yang Qi to head inward to move stagnation, making the child more susceptible to the invasion of pathogenic factors since Wei Qi is less available to the exterior (Wei Qi being a subset of Yang Qi).

---

1. The measurements are not to be confused with Wen Bing diagnosis at ST-9 where one inquires about the width of the pulse.

CHILDREN AND THE EIGHT EXTRAORDINARY CHANNEL PULSES

During this time bonding with the mother is the primary importance, the principal reality of a healthy child. Normally during the first three years we don't examine pulses at the radial artery, relying instead upon the index finger, as mentioned above. However, wrist pulses are often readable at the time a child begins walking. If you were to read the radial pulses of a two year old, you would likely find moving pulses that float up through all three levels, demonstrating the evolving Du Mai Channel. These pulses should be floating but not rapid or tight. This is considered harmonious and healthy. The child is beginning to separate from the mother and gain some independence by walking.

Ren Mai gives birth to Du Mai and then Du gives birth to all the other channels. One way to understand how Ren and Du give birth to Chong and the other Extraordinary Channels in turn is through understanding the inner responses children make while progressively encountering the world. In the process of developing—experiencing and exploring the world—the child will eventually encounter the word "no." Limitations are encountered and the child feels love is conditional since the latitude granted to do as they please is withdrawn. These limits stimulate the child to focus strongly on what they want. This causes the retrieval of Yang, bringing it into the moderate level and into Chong Mai. Chong is the Sea of Postnatal Qi and absorbs the information related to parental guidance and direction along with the learning of submission as the child adjusts to the Postnatal environment. At this point of development, as the child is learning to temper and maintain self-control, the child presents with a Chong Mai pulse. If the Chong pulse is not tight, this process is going well.

If the parents are doting, overstimulating the child with too many toys, too much noise, too many colors, trying make up for what they themselves didn't have, Du Mai may behave pathologically and hyperactivity disorders can develop. These children have relatively strong floating pulses in all three positions and through all three levels, but they are pathological in that they are wiry; the child is "wired". They cannot seem to find fulfillment because they are never allowed to be Yin.

Ren Mai and Chong Mai can be disorientated by vaccinations. The Ren is affected directly by a vaccine because the Yin of the Ren—The Sea of Yin—is the mediumship for latency of the vaccine. (Vaccines are designed to reach as deeply into the system as possible for long-lasting effect, essentially being designed for the level of latency.) This is the mechanism for keeping it away from the organs. Vaccines are administered at the very time Ren Mai is most active and responsive and this serves to magnify the effect of this very strong pathogenic factor. If the child has weak Jing, more Yin must be allocated for the latency of the vaccine.

The greater the amount of Yin called upon to provide latency, the lower the child's capacity to engender Yang Qi. This is because Yang Qi is responsible for holding the pathogen in place within the Yin. Yang is too taxed and cannot be correctly articulated. Yin becomes out of balance and Yin activity becomes constant. The Ren Mai pulse is tight. This is the mechanism of neurodevelopmental disorders.

It would be incorrect to disperse Ren Mai because that is the body's safety mechanism. Ideally this is dealt with preemptively in utero. Needling and moxaing KI-9 at the end of each trimester to assist the fetus in releasing fire toxins acquired in utero somewhat lessens the burden placed on the immune system postnatally. In the KI-9 treatment, Yin Wei Mai is supporting Ren Mai. Bao Mai is also an option after birth since the vaccine was introduced to the Blood.

This is all happening at a time the Chong is developing. Chong appears as a relatively healthy pulse after the child has weaned, achieved the upright posture, gone out into the world, is assimilating external food and engaging in relationships within and outside the family. The Chong is highly influenced by external and social stimulus, for example, pre-school. The role of the Chong is to foster the child's discovery of their own body, and to begin to receive stimulation and form perceptions about the world. The child learns how other people live and how they react to authority. The child takes that information and begins to experiment with boundaries in their relationships with their parents, with others and with the environment.

The entire process of dealing with major pathogens adversely affects Chong Mai as it acts to mediate between Ren and Du, balancing Yin and Yang. If the Chong is busy dealing with the impact of toxins introduced to it, or if the child is confused by too much input from people and environments not within the bounds of the developing child's sanctuary, imbalances can occur in this phase of development. The child's alignment with the outside world is skewed. The Chong pulse will emerge with tightness in it.

Note: While the Eight Extra Channels can be used in children of this age, DU-4 is strictly contraindicated before the completion of puberty. Needle children very sparingly; they are highly responsive to acupuncture. Two carefully chosen points are usually adequate.

THE ROOT OF THE MOUNTAIN

The area between the eyes, across the bridge of the nose but below the third eye is known as the Mountain Gate, The Root of the Mountain, or The Health Palace. Often a colored vein will become visible in this area. It is an important site of diagnosis prior to the age of three. Newborns often have this vein showing because their digestion is not yet strong. The vein's visibility should dissipate after nine months. Its presence is not expected at all after eighteen months.

Babies under three months of age are very Yin. They have not begun to articulate Yang Qi. In babies of this age, there should not be a purple or crimson vein on the finger or the Root of the Mountain. After three months, Yin goes into relative decline and Yang becomes exuberant. Fevers arise from the exuberance of the Du Channel and can be very high.

If the amount of food given is not moderate, is not very regular, and the child is instead given very large meals or forced to eat, the Kidneys are not allowed to develop at a steady rate and hives or skin conditions can erupt. Babies are adept at regulating their own intake.

A green vein at the Root of the Mountain indicates a deficiency of Spleen Qi. More regular, smaller feedings are required to reduce pressure on the Spleen. Food intolerances develop early if the Spleen is stagnated. The amount fed can be reduced dramatically if the frequency of feeding increases in kind. In severe cases, tiny amounts can be given at 20 minute intervals.

If the vein at the Root is blue there is a Kidney Yang deficiency, or Cold. The child must be covered, especially around the neck so as not to develop respiratory allergies.

THE EAR

Examine the right ear in girls, the left in boys. Look for nodules, prominent and engorged veins. Nodules in the ears indicate stagnation of Kidney Yin. If the Kidney Yin is stagnant, it cannot anchor Kidney Yang. The child may not be grounded and may have trouble sleeping because the Yang of the Kidney is escaping. Points on the Ren Channel would be chosen to support Kidney Yin, to consolidate the Yin. If there is a red vein in the Life Gate of the finger and you also find a pulse at SI-19, Internal Heat is being expressed and must be cleared.

YIN TANG

Also called Ming Tang, The Bright Hall, or The Third Eye, the area just above where the eyebrows would meet should have a certain shine, brightness or lustre, because the spirit is expressed there. In children this area should be shiny as a result of their abundant Qi. If the area is flaky, there is Lung Qi deficiency. If child has blue discoloration between the eyebrows, the Lungs are unable to control the Liver due to stagnation and perhaps Cold.

Wind disturbances are likely in this scenario. If there are blue veins at Yin Tang and the child is crying a lot, there is pain. Use Xi-Cleft points to relieve it.

Children can see things we adults can no longer see. They have not yet yielded to society's agreements about limitations to perception. If Yin Tang is overly active they may need help integrating with society. If there is redness present, the Shen is disturbed; the child is affected by internal Heat. The cause of this Heat could result from a range of things from soy milk to overstimulation. Children's rooms should be one soothing color and toys should be few and not passively generate their own sounds.

Heat from the Root of the Mountain can work its way up to Ming Tang. If you find a green vein extending from the Root of the Mountain toward Ming Tang, the Spleen is unable to adequately store Blood. The child's capacity for concentration is adversely affected by too much stimulation. This is the early manifestation of ADHD (Attention Deficiency Hyperactivity Disorder). The Spleen cannot bank enough Blood to enable the child to make sense of what is being experienced. The diet needs to change to strengthen the Spleen and allow it to bank Blood. Sugar should be eliminated. Dairy (not including butter) and gluten should at the very least be greatly lowered. Lotus seeds (pureed) are a principal food here as they calm the Shen and allow the Spleen to bank Blood.

CHAPTER 11

PULSE TAKING DURING TREATMENT

It's imperative to take pulses before, during and after treatment. There's no better barometer of the correctness of your diagnosis, the progress of the treatment, the efficacy of the sequence of its execution, and the body's response to the treatment. Taking the pulses during treatment alerts you to the need to change tack, to add another point, to take a needle out and indicates the conclusion of the treatment (as the pulses indicate the intended change). It's important to know if a different course need be taken from the outset, to admit one's diagnosis or strategy is incorrect.

Conversely, there might be a quiet, spontaneous healing which allows you to progress to the next treatment immediately. Taking the pulses during treatment allows you to be truly in the moment. This is a reason it's not prudent to spell out exactly what you plan to do in the session before you start. It's far more in line with the spirit of what we do to begin the treatment, check the pulses to ascertain whether the Qi is moving as you expect it to (or better) but be ready to find that it is actually not and that a change in plan is needed.

PATIENT CONFIDENCE IN THE PRACTITIONER

It used to be that a patient visiting an acupuncturist would not say anything about the complaint but simply hold out their wrist, knowing the practitioner would find everything pertinent. Whether or not you had to tell the acupuncturist your complaint was a marker of whether the practitioner was competent or not. Of course part of that was cultural when people were unwilling to discuss processes of the Lower Jiao, but the underlying idea was that practitioners should be able not only to feel the issue in the pulses but also should be able to see more about it than can be described in common language. These days, with the interest in detailed pulse diagnosis rapidly increasing and the rising public interest in acupuncture, more patients are expecting good pulse reading.

The act of taking pulses after the patient sits down serves to orientate the patient to the treatment. As you describe what you are finding you are initiating the treatment. The treatment has already started. During the process of taking the pulses the practitioner reports the way in which the pulses are changing. The patient will feel change in the movement of Qi before the treatment has begun.

If you are new to a detailed pulse method, it may be helpful to note that there are certain

190

things that are easy to find in the pulse and that when reported to the patient increase their confidence in your abilities. These observations can even open the way for the patient to trust the practitioner in quite a profound way.

The first thing I look for is tight, superficial pulses. If you learn the pulse map of the Sinew channels and the anatomy they represent, which is an easy straight-forward study, you can estimate with confidence where pain, stiffness, or tension is in the body. For example, if the cun position has a tight, superficial pulse and/or slightly rapid pulse, there is Wind-Cold trapped in the Tai Yang sinews. The rapidity implies that the tightness is sitting in the superior regions of those two Sinews and that the body is beginning to respond with Hear. You could say, "It seems as though there is some tightness in your shoulders or the back or your neck". The patient will either agree or say, "I've been getting headaches at the back of my head," or something like that.

Another easy thing to find is dehydration. If the moderate level of the right guan is thin, narrow or small, if it has very little width, there are insufficient Stomach Fluids. You could suggest that the patient is dehydrated. The patient will either agree or will say they do drink a lot of water. You will know they are not retaining fluids and are urinating frequently. (They need wet foods, not just water.)

Also simple to deduce is lack of deep sleep or lack of early sleep. If the Kidney Yin pulse is felt in the superficial level, there is some sleep disturbance. If the Liver pulse is at the same time tight and superficial, there's tossing and turning. If the Heart pulse is at the same time empty, there is trouble falling asleep.

These are just a few of the many ways the pulses speak volumes about the patient. Allow the pulses to speak for themselves. If you can find the information, the patient wants you to have it.

After a long period of practice you will become so comfortable with the method that you will find yourself identifying in the pulses things you perhaps had not considered could be there. The patient might think the whole thing miraculous, wondering how so much detail could possibly be seen, but good pulse taking is very logical and very learnable. Only practice is required.

TAKING PULSES WHILE RELEASING THE EXTERIOR

If you find tight, superficial pulses, it's important to release the exterior before you go on to other treatment. Blockages in the Wei level impede the free flow of Qi. Perhaps you might choose to do sliding cups, gua sha, a Sinew treatment. During a Sinew treatment repeated checking of the pulse saves time. Instead of releasing the Wei level all the way along the Channel, palpate to find the tightness, release it with the technique you've chosen and then go back to the pulse to see whether the entire channel is now released. A tight pulse will become harmonized the instant the channel releases.

During abdominal palpation and needling to release stagnation, consult the pulses to determine whether you have fully released abdominal blockages. Go back and check to see whether the pulse has harmonized. Checking the pulse enables the practitioner to minimize the number of needles used.

CHECKING THE TREATMENT STRATEGY

The pulses will show the effect of your treatment strategy immediately after the needles have been set. If you clear Heat, for example, the pulse will immediately slow down. If you break up Cold, the pulse will immediately speed up. If you clear Dampness, the pulse will immediately be less slippery. Taking pulses right after you're finished inserting needles is key in ascertaining whether the method or the point you chose is working for that individual.

If you clear Heat during a treatment and another pulse becomes rapid, you merely shifted the Heat somewhere else. It did not clear. If you moxa a certain channel to scatter Cold and another pulse then becomes superficially tight, the Sinew Channels are bringing that Cold to the surface for release to the exterior. That Sinew must be released for the initial treatment to be successful. The patient could leave in pain otherwise. A patient should not leave in new pain.

If you are treating pathology related to hidden pulses—for example, the Divergent or Eight Extra Channels—often during or after the treatment the pulses will no longer be moving pulses. They will have harmonized and become steady. This does not always happen but when it doesn't happen it does not mean that the treatment was not successful.

CHECKING PULSES NEAR THE END OF TREATMENT

After the treatment has fully settled in, check the pulses again to see if the pulses have the desired change. For example, if you do a Dai Mai treatment and find that even after the treatment has been in 30 minutes, the pulses are still slippery (indicating Dampness is being retained) add moxa to the treatment. Moxa the needles. If the pulses become rapid as the patient retains Heat, you might bleed a Luo point or plum blossom where Heat is accumulating. If the Dai Mai becomes Cold, you could moxa the entire area. If you find the pulses wiry, you might palpate the Mu points and release those. You might release the He Sea points to release the bowels to help drain, since Dai Mai, your chosen treatment, is being stubborn. The point is that if the pulses are not checked none of these adjustments can be determined accurately and the patient feels that the treatment didn't really make the grade.

END OF TREATMENT PULSE CHECK

At the end of a treatment the change in direction you are seeking should be evident in the pulses. Actually, it's a lot of fun to check the pulses after the treatment because the picture after a properly constructed treatment is extraordinary. It's constant confirmation that you're making a significant contribution in providing an arena for the change the patient is enacting.

At the end of the treatment, it's very potent to be able to report to the patient the changes that you are observing in the pulses, explaining that there has been positive change. This communication, even if not spoken, is important to healing.

A question I am very often asked is how is it possible for pulses to be noticeably wider after the treatment. How can this happen since the patient didn't eat, drink or sleep during the treatment? The pulses show evidence of the body's comprehension of your intention. There can be marked change in pulses without nourishment or sleep being added. When this happens after treatment, it means that the body is understanding the intention of the treatment and responding by signaling a feeling of repleteness. It's almost as though the body is sighing with relief. If, for example, the intention of the treatment had been to nourish Blood, the patient may feel hungry, thirsty and more tired because the treatment has shifted the body into nourishment mode to meet the invitation set into the pulse. (This tiredness is not pathological, but essential for the assimilation of nourishment, and repair.)

THE RATE OF CHANGE IN THE PULSES IN TREATMENT

If you are treating a functional change, that is, the way in which a Channel conducts Qi, the changes in the pulses can occur quite quickly. If you are treating organ dysfunction, that is, pathology of the organ itself not just its channel, the changes during and after treatment will still be significant, but the entire healing process will be slower. Likewise, in diagnosis, if you can change the pulse by willing the pulse to change, the issue is in the channel. If you cannot will the pulse to change, the issue is in the organ itself.

THE MOST IMPORTANT THING

The most important thing is not to focus on treating signs and symptoms. Base your diagnosis on your pulse findings. The signs and symptoms are simply a way for the patient to communicate discomfort to you. Taking pulses and making diagnoses from them is the single most potent way to build your practice because you will consistently be treating the root of the disease. If you treat a headache, you might or might not have a successful session. (Success being defined as prolonged increased freedom experienced by the patient.) If the patient presents with a headache and you find that the Liver pulse is thin, build Blood. Building Blood addresses the systemic scenario from which the headache is arising. If a patient presents with a sore knee and you treat that sore knee, you might get some relief for a few days or you might not. But if you find that there's a Bladder Divergent pulse, or a Stomach Sinew pulse, or even just a Yin deficiency or a Yang deficiency and treat that, you are treating the systemic issue that led to that sore knee. Then and only then, treat the knee locally. That could be done in the same session.

APPENDIX I

THE TRIPLE HEATER PULSE

The pulses of the chi position (the Kidney pulses) should be deep, rounded, strong, relaxed and contained within the deep level. Occasionally the right chi pulse will be found in the moderate level. When this happens, it is usually tight. This is called a Pericardium pulse; the pericardium is tightening in order to protect the Heart. Sometimes the right chi pulse is found in the superficial level, indicating a Sinew issue. And sometimes the right chi pulse is found to float to the superficial level, indicating escaping Yang. This usually means there is insufficient Yin to contain Kidney Yang. Since the Yang is not anchored down it is free to rise and will follow your finger, floating up into the superficial level of the pulse.

On rare occasions the Kidney pulse can be quite rapid and follow your finger up, almost pushing your finger with an accompanying fullness through the deep and moderate levels and then all the way through the superficial level to the point where it feels as if it is protruding above the level of the skin, remaining rapid throughout. This is called a Triple Heater pulse. Such a pulse is not to be confused with a floating Yang pulse. The Triple Heater pulse has an urgency about it and sits very high in the pulse. This pulse indicates a loss of latency; the body is unable to hold a pathogen latent (hidden) any longer and is releasing a pathogen from the Jing-Essence. The pathogen has a fiery nature and has been causing inflammation that has affected the integrity of the Jing. What you are feeling in the pulse is the release of fire toxins. In Western terms this could be thought of as an overrun of free radicals (a precancerous condition, corruption of the DNA, or worse).

The *Mai Jing* says that these pulses indicate some type of decay or consumption of the flesh that can eventually lead to death. The Heat is understood to be coming from the constitutional level, from the organs, from Yang Ming where Heat originates, or from the interface of the Primary Channels and the organs.

The fullness underneath this pulse that pushes it up from the deep level indicates that it is coming up from that deep level. This is how we know that the pulse does not reflect the presence of an external pathogenic factor.

STRONG AND WEAK TRIPLE HEATER PULSES
The body's complement of Jing-Essence is reflected deep in the Kidney pulses. Essence is the commodity from which Yin and Yang are made. To enact a successful clearing of toxins from the Yuan level, there must be both Yang Qi to push the toxin out and Yin to

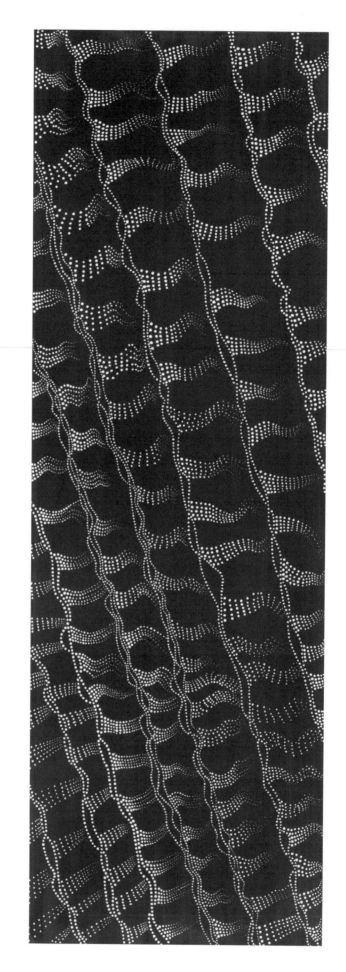

The Triple Heater Pulse

Triple Heater Pulse, found in the right chi position if present, indicates a state of lost latency. The body has lost the ability to hold pathology away from the organs in the Luo Channels or the joints (Divergent Channels). The heat of the formerly contained pathology spills up and out in an uncontrolled and wild display. The pulse is very rapid and with every beat, pushes the practitioner's finger steadily upward, then seemingly beyond the surface of the patient's skin.

provide mediumship to transport the toxin. If you press down deeply into this pulse and don't feel anything pushing back at your finger and the pulse is thin, it means that there's a deficiency of Jing-Essence, that the capacity to generate both Yin and Yang at the Yuan level is weak. Upright Qi is weak. If the pulse pushes back at you at the deep level but is thin, willingness to activate the Triple Heater mechanism is there but there isn't enough Jing-Essence to drive it. Cultivation is required to rebuild the Triple Heater mechanism: meditation, qigong, some kind of activity. Treatments to accompany this cultivation could include TH-4, Pooling of Yang, to build its Qi, LI-4 and LI-6 to regulate Fluids, and ST-37 and ST-39 to regulate blood.

When taking the Triple Heater pulse, note its status. After you've determined there is a Triple Heater pulse, if you press slowly back down into the Yuan level and find strength there—a strong sense of the pulse pressing up against your finger and the pulse with good width—the body is engaged in a healing crisis. It is potentially successful in pushing fire toxins out of the Jing. Use the Divergent Channels to assist the body in moving those fire toxins up from the Jing to the Wei level.

However, after you've determined there is a floating Triple Heater pulse, if you press slowly back down into the Yuan level and find the pulse weak at the deep level with no real pressure up against your finger, there is a deficiency of Jing-Essence. The body has lost latency and fire toxins are leaking out of the Jing. This is not a healing crisis but a plain crisis. The fire toxins cannot be cleared by the body or cleared in treatment because there is insufficient Qi to mount an attempt to move the toxins out. Any effort to do so will result in increased auto-intoxication, a dangerous scenario. Use the Eight Extra Channels to assist the body in retaining the toxins and to maximize the body's capacity to regain latency while you assist the body in building back the Yin that will be needed to eradicate the toxins when the body is capable.

When a Triple Heater pulse is found, a clinical decision must be made—whether to clear the fire toxin condition or to support latency by keeping the condition quiet and away from the organs while the system is strengthened enough to be able to clear the condition at a later date. (This is roughly equivalent to remission in Western medicine.) If the Triple Heater pulse is strong and wide, work to clear the condition, but if the Triple Heater pulse is weak or thin, work to create and support latency. This is the work of the Divergent Channels, usually the fourth confluence.

LEFT AND RIGHT FLOATING PULSES

Pericardium, floating Yang, and Triple Heater pulses can be found in either the right or the left pulses. Pericardium and Triple Heater pulses, however, are usually found on the right wrist because that is their elemental position in the pulse arena. Triple Heater is generally associated with the right wrist. Floating Yang pulses are found equally on either wrist.

CONCLUSIVENESS OF THE TRIPLE HEATER FLOATING PULSE

The absence of a Triple Heater pulse is not conclusive in determining the absence of a fire toxin condition. Many times I have seen fire toxin conditions with no Triple Heater pulses. In two of those cases, there was no hint of a Triple Heater pulse (though very weak Jing-Essence) and yet the patients had been diagnosed with second and fourth stage cancers. I later came to realize that the body was so overwhelmed with the condition that it was not capable of trying to release the toxins and there was insufficient Qi to raise the pulse of the Triple Heater. The condition had become overwhelming in each case. In another case, the patient had a self-destructive wish and the fire toxin condition provided the much sought after back door exit to life. The mind was preventing action by the Triple Heater mechanism. The psychology of fire toxin diseases is important enough to be the subject of a text of its own.

ASPECTS OF LATENCY OF A PATHOGENIC FACTOR

1. If the Sinews fail, the pathogen moves either to the Divergent or to the Luo Channels. When those avenues are exhausted, the Eight Extra Channels can absorb the pathology. When a pathogen is being held latent in the Luos, Divergents or Eight Extras, there are no signs or symptoms.

2. If the Tai Yang Sinew—the very first line of defense for an external pathogenic factor—fails and the Luo Channels do not absorb the pathogen, the pathogen can enter the He-Sea point of the Bladder Primary Channel. The body diverts the pathogen from the Bladder organ (to which the He-Sea has access) to the joints. The pathogen has entered the Divergent Channel sequence at that point.

3. If the Luo Channels are taxed due to Ying (Blood or Fluid) deficiency, the pathogen can go to the Divergent Channels.

4. If the Sinews fail due to insufficient Yang, the pathogen can go to the joints. As Jing declines, latency is lost (symptoms emerge as the pathogen becomes unhidden in the joints) and arthritis ensues.

5. If Ying is taxed by heat, the Jing may step in and use its cold to hold the pathogen. When latency is lost from the Jing, heat along with the pathology is released, causing the Triple Heater pulse to float as it tries to clear the Jing of pathology. The pathogen

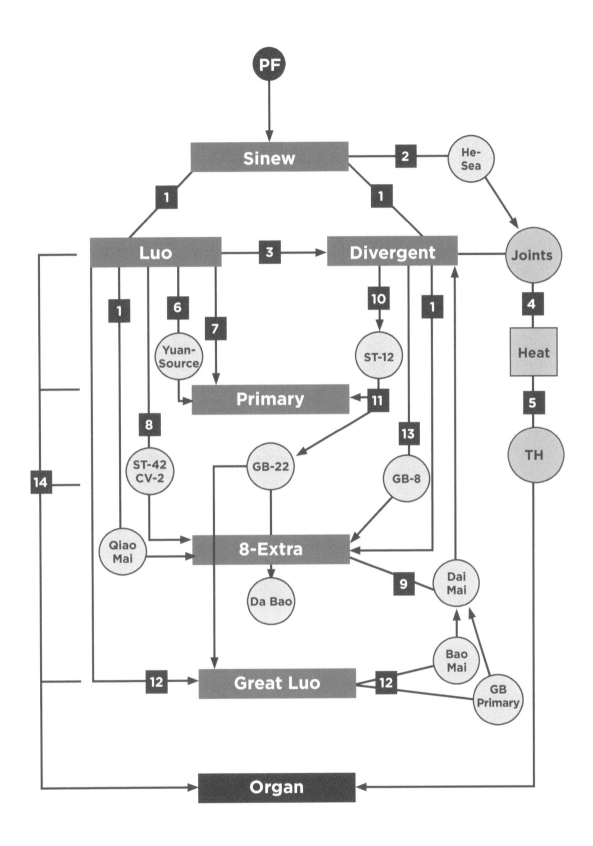

The Triple Heater pulse is often found when the entire channel system has failed to maintain latency of a pathogenic factor. The body's mechanisms for latency are described in this diagram.

then has access to the organs. Therefore the body will try at all costs to find an alternative reservoir of latency.

6. The Luo Channels can empty into the Yuan-Source level if they overflow with pathology and fail to find a neighboring Luo to occupy.

7. The Luos can empty into their related Primary Channel or a neighboring Luo.

8. Pathology in the Luos can find its way to the Eight Extra Channels. The last Yang Luo (the Gallbladder Luo) can empty its pathology to ST-42 which connects to Chong Mai, and the last Yin Luo (the Liver Luo) can empty into the Ren Mai at the end of its trajectory, CV-2, giving entry to the Constitution.

9. The Constitution can pass the pathology to its main reservoir, Dai Mai. When Dai Mai fills, it should drain, but if it cannot, it uses Kidney Divergent Channel to extend its field of latency.

10. Once in a Divergent Channel, the pathogen can then move through the Divergent Channel sequence until it reaches the last confluence, the Large Intestine and Lung Divergent Channels.

11. At the end of the Divergent Channel sequence, the pathogen can enter the Primary Channels at ST-12, but the body may try to push the pathology to the Da Bao at GB-22 which is another point on the Lung Divergent Channel trajectory. GB-22 is also the Great Luo of the Spleen and the pathogen can find latency in the Luo arena there, also.

12. When The Great Luo of the Spleen fills, the pathology can spill down via either the GB Primary Channel or Bao Mai to Dai Mai, a major holding site.

13. At the end of the Divergent Channel sequence, the pathogen can go to Du Mai at GB-8.

14. When the capacity to hold the pathogen in latency is exhausted, the pathogen moves to the organs and the disease becomes terminal.

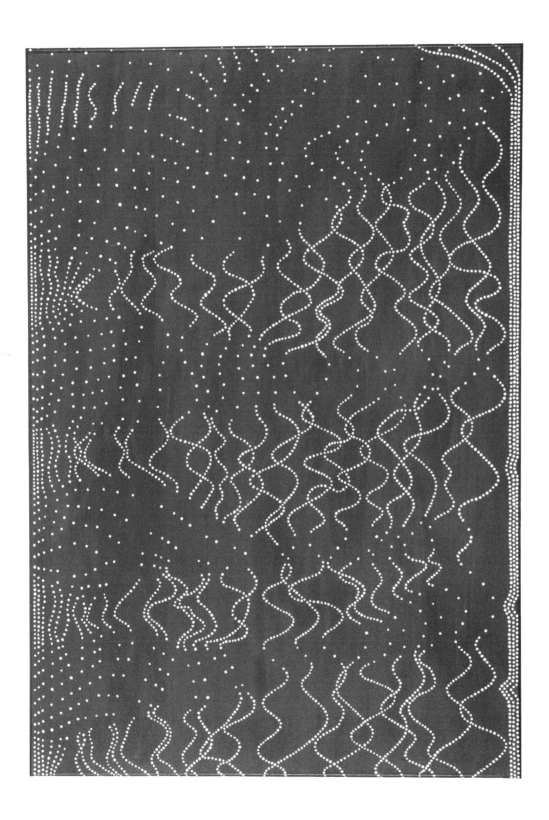

Transition

This work depicts the emotional palette reflected in the pulse during treatment of a terminal illness. Knowledge of the disease, which shows as a corruption in the smooth flow of Constitutional Qi in the lowest part of the painting, creates havoc in the Heart as the person struggles with the idea that they may die, while trying desperately to stay afloat. The emotions, shown in the wavy lines, become constrained and torqued. The immune system, shown in the top quarter, breaks down as Wei Qi scatters. Ultimately, the emotions dissolve, heart-to-heart and eye-to-eye contact is lost and there is only pain. Latency of the pathogenic factor is lost. Constitutional Qi which cradles life evaporates, and the spirit is released to the ethers. This painting was made during the last three days of my father's life as I held his hand and pulse, trying my best to comfort him.

APPENDIX II

QUESTIONS AND DISCUSSION

The questions in this section are loosely organized in the following way:

GENERAL QUESTIONS

Often I find that the guan position is floating but the cun is not. Is this a problem?

Yes, this is telling you the pathology is trapped. Release the exterior and allow the exterior to express the pathology outward. The Jing-Well and the Luo points can perform this function.

I always find a mixture of excess and deficient pulses. Is this expected?

Yes, if there is a deficiency somewhere, there will be an excess to compensate somewhere else and vice versa. Deficiency or excess without compensation by other organs or media would indicate very serious cases, where the body is no longer able to activate an attempt to balance.

Why do I often feel that the right pulses are so much stronger than the left pulses?

The two wrists reflect the dynamics of pathology and resistance to pathology. Yin and Yang are constantly balancing and transforming into one another. Because the right side of the body is Yin, it is trying to move toward being Yang. The right wrist reflects the way in which the body is using its Yang to push pathology out.

The left side of the body is Yang, so it is trying to move toward being Yin. Yang resides at the surface, so the left side reflects the way in which the body is using its Qi in the form of humors to gather Qi back down and in.

Therefore, on the right as you press down you should feel things pushing out. There should be a discernible resistance in each of the positions of the right wrist. This tells you there is enough fluid to clear a pathogen. The exocrine fluids which are a subset of Jin-Thin fluids are used by the Lungs and Stomach to carry pathology out of the body. The Lungs release pathogens through sweating or, later, coughing. The Sinew Channels cannot function to release pathology without these Jin-Thin Fluids. By thinning Phlegm with Fluids the Spleen transforms the Dampness that enables pathology to linger in the body. The Stomach must be ready to vomit out a pathogen. The Kidneys disinhibit pathogens through the urine. Triple Heater must be equipped to push pathology out of the Yuan level. All these functions are outward and show as such in the pulse.

On the left wrist as you press down you should feel a retreating, a feeling of receiving, a cushiony feeling as a reflection of the body's capacity to hold pathology in latency.

The left pulses consolidate. The Kidneys govern latency at the Yuan level which then becomes the provenance of the Eight Extraordinary Channels. This also tells you there are enough fluids to maintain the integrity of the structure. The Bladder controls the Sinews which are responsible for holding pathology latent in the sinews. The Gallbladder Channel brings things back into the bone for latency. (The Jia Yi Jing says the Gallbladder controls the bone.) The Small Intestine is the first channel of latency in the Primary Channel sequence. Further, SI-18 is the confluent point of the sinews which we needle to release latency there.

The individual positions on each side must be felt with the feeling of releasing or of holding kept in mind. The Large Intestine manages Jin-Thin Fluids, and since the status of those Fluids is shown in the width of the right cun position, that position should push out slightly. The Small Intestine manages Ye-Thick Fluids and is shown in the width of the left cun position. Under pressure that position should relax inward slightly.

What does it mean if the pulses on both sides push back at your finger?
If both sides push back out, it means the person has difficulty being in the mode of receiving and has overextended him or her self. If the pulses are floating and thin, there is insufficient Blood and/or Fluids.

Why do the left pulses often feel weak?
The natural retreating quality in the left side should not be mistaken for a weaker pulse. What we are feeling is simply that the sides are reflecting the interplay of Yin and Yang: the left retreats inward while the right expresses outward.

Why am I finding in some women that the left pulses push back at my finger?
During menstruation the body is not in the mode of receiving because the body is purging Blood. During that time, if you push down on the superficial level of the pulses they can seem to be pushing back up rather than giving way to your pressure and revealing their receptive nature. This would not be the time for a treatment to consolidate. The body is more interested in consolidation at mid-cycle.

What should I do if the right pulses are not subtly pushing out?

If the right pulses in general do not give the feeling they are at least subtly pushing out, an aspect of the diagnosis must address that. The possible reasons for the lack of push are numerous. There could be blockages, deficient Qi, deficient Fluids, deficient Yang, etc.

What should I do if the left pulses are not subtly receiving?

If the left side in general does not give the feeling of receiving, an aspect of the diagnosis must reflect that. Commonly the reason for this is a lack of some kind of mediumship: Jin-Thin or Ye-Thick Fluids, Blood or Jing. Often a person with these pulses has a hard time receiving; they give too much of themselves and overextend themselves. The Eight Extras address this quite beautifully.

What does it mean if the left pulses are trying to push back at my finger?

It means that the Ye-Thick Fluids, Blood or the Jing are trying to expel something pathological.

If the left pulses are floating and the right is not, what should I do?

If the left side is floating and the right is not, Yang is exiting. Hydrate by nourishing Fluids.

Why are conditions considered severe when the pathology is found in the left pulses?

The left side reflects severity because the condition is being kept latent or trapped at a deeper level by Yin, Dampness, Jing or Blood.

On the left side, when I press down just below the Ying level, the pulse gets softer and almost melts into the bone level. What does this mean?

It means that postnatal Qi is being transformed into prenatal Qi, or that the body has the capacity to hold a pathogen latent.

My patient's pulses are consolidating on the right and pushing out on the left; the sides are the opposite of what we would expect. What should I do?

This could be a polarity issue. If so, treat it with the four gates or the inner four gates; LI-4 and LR-3 or LU-1 and LR-14.

Is there a way to think about the two wrists being connected?

The non-pathological movement of Qi goes up on the left and down on the right. The Kidney pulse on the left side should be deep because Yin is stored at the Yuan level and is meted out with conservation. The Heart pulse is naturally slightly scattered because Yin is drawn upward from the Kidney to the Liver as Yang is moved upward into the Heart. The

Liver pulse is healthy when it is slightly tight because at this point the Liver is still holding on to Yin and Blood. The Heart Blood is propelled by Lung Qi. It must connect across to the Lungs on the right where the Lungs float to gather, harvest and consolidate Qi and draw it back down to the deep level. (Lung Qi fans Ming Men fire.) The Spleen pulse is healthy when it is relaxed as digestion needs to be relaxed. The Qi then moves into the right Kidney via Triple Heater to conserve and consolidate since the right side is Yin. The Kidney pulse therefore is healthy when it is latent, like a stone.

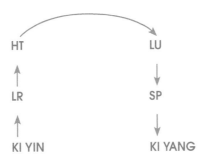

This is not to be confused with the quest for latency or eradication of a pathogen where we see the left pulses providing the mediumship for latency and the right pulses reflecting the adequacy of Qi to move a pathogen out.

Is it possible to determine by the pulses whether a condition is chronic?
Chronic conditions are indicated by the presence of floating-long or floating-scattered pulses.

Does a narrow pulse always mean that there is a deficiency?
A true deficiency occurs when there is an absence of width together with failure to consolidate that medium. Consolidation is affirmed when you press into a left wrist pulse and it yields to pressure, softening and giving in to your finger. Consolidation should not be confused with weakness.

When I take pulses it seems that the width changes between the superficial, moderate and deep levels. The moderate level can appear narrow under the finger while the deep level feels wide. How can this happen when anatomically the radial artery is narrower at the deep level?
The three levels of the pulse are resonators. They resonate or echo the state of the entire being. When you examine the width, the densest Qi will be reflected in the lowest level of the pulse. The width you're feeling has little to do with the artery itself; it's merely a resonance, a vibration that's picked up from the mediumship related to that level and exhibiting in the pulse. The Ying level humors will resonate with the middle of the pulse. The Wei level will resonate with the superficial level of the pulse; it has nothing to do with the fact that you might

be palpating well above the height of the radial artery. Hence, the three depths can be entirely different widths. The moderate level can theoretically be narrower than the other two levels.

Are there aspects of the entire being I will not be able to determine from the pulse?

The pulses give the entire state of the individual. The only limitations to what a patient's pulses can convey arise from the practitioner's knowledge, expectations and cultivation. What the pulses offer is so complete that traditionally very skilled practitioners deliberately choose not to read certain aspects of that information because they philosophically believe certain connections within a life are not for others to investigate.

How is it possible for the pulses to be at differing tempos?

Each pulse position reflects an organ's unique properties and each organ's individual pathology. If there is Heat in the Stomach, the vibration emanating from the Stomach that then comes through the Stomach Channel and lands at the relay station that is the pulse of the Stomach (right guan position) will vibrate (beat) at a relatively high tempo; it will be rapid. If, concurrently there is Cold in the Lungs, the vibration that is emanating from the Lungs, through the Lung Channel and into the relay station that is the Lung pulse (right cun) will beat at a relatively slow tempo. This can happen concurrently because the two organs are in very different states. What we feel in the pulse is the vibrations of all the organs, distributed by the grand circulator, the Heart. The best way to come to understanding of this is through experience. As you find pulses at differing tempos and you diagnose them clearly and treat the patient successfully, true confidence arises in the system.

Can a pulse change when one single needle is inserted?

Yes, certainly. And they do. They can change without a needle, too. The causative factor is the intention of the practitioner. (Incidentally, one needle does not create a treatment. You need at least two. Qi is relationship.)

When I am taking pulses, sometimes I'll find a tight or wiry quality but then when I ask a question about it, the pulse relaxes immediately. How can this happen when I haven't needled yet?

The simple act of bringing a patient's awareness to the parts or aspects of their body that needs balancing also brings their focus to the tension itself. Once tension becomes registered in consciousness, it needs consciousness to maintain it and that takes effort. It's easier for the patient to let it go than to harbor it.

We heard about having a dialogue with the pulses. How can I generate a Yuan level pulse if it's missing?

You would press into the bone with 15 beans of pressure and have a dialogue there. Release pressure to 14 beans every now and then and see if the bone is willing to generate a pulse for you. It may take a little while.

What is the significance of the pulse at ST-42?

If LU-9 is tight and superficial and you determine that there's an external pathogenic factor, palpate ST-42. If you find that ST-42 is floating but empty, there is insufficient Kidney Yang to support Wei Qi in its efforts to produce a purge.

Should I practice taking pulses at GB-3, KI-3, ST-9, ST-42 and BL-60?

If you're interested in them. These pulses were once used to ascertain whether there was a problem in an organ after something pathological was found in the deep level of the pulses. If the deep level of the Lung pulse showed pathology, GB-3 was palpated and if found floating, confirmed a problem in the Lung organ. If the deep level of the Heart pulse showed pathology, KI-3 was palpated and if found floating confirmed a problem in the Pericardium, Triple Heater, Heart organ or perhaps the Kidney organ.

If the Small or Large Intestine pulses were found to be pathological, particularly long, firm or scattered, comparisons were made at ST-9. If the pulse at ST-9 was twice as big as the pulse at LU-9 on the right hand, the condition was understood to be in Shao Yang. If it was three times bigger than LU-9 it was thought to be in Tai Yang. If it was four times bigger than LU-9, the condition had moved to Yang Ming. ST-42 was used to measure how well Yang Qi is supporting Wei Qi. If you found a floating pulse at ST-42 and, as you pressed down into it, found it weak or empty, it would mean that the patient had a Wei level condition that could become chronic if not treated since they didn't have the support of Yang Qi. The issue was treated at the Middle Jiao organs: the Spleen, Stomach, Liver or Gallbladder. If you found pathology at the left chi position and a floating pulse at BL-60, there was thought to be pathology in the Kidney or Bladder organ.

How do pulses change during a healing crisis?

A healing crisis is a short illness during which the body finally purges latent pathology. Pulses are not tight in a healing crisis and can even become remarkably relaxed.

How are the pulse positions viewed in a philosophical sense?

The floating pulse represents heaven's Qi, the spirit or the Shen taking up residence in the Heart. The Lungs reach up to heaven as they release the exterior. Both cun positions should float as Qi is expressed outwardly by the Lungs and by the Shen which is contained in the Blood. Every human should have floating pulses at the cun position because everyone should be expressing their Qi and Blood, with no holding back. These pulses indicate joy in life and a willingness to share it. On inhalation, the floating pulse in the cun indicates the patient is assimilating the forces of Heaven. Heaven joins us through our breath, enters the channels and animates the Blood to animate life. As you push down at the superior level of the Heart, you feel that the Heart is receiving celestial Qi and moving it inward. Heavenly Qi seeps into the bone to illuminate the Jing-Essence so that we can see our own destiny, so we can see what our life is about. You should be able to create a floating pulse in the cun position if there isn't one already. If you can't, the patient is unable to receive inspiration, adapt to change, or there's a blockage.

If both pulses are pushing up, the patient has a difficult time receiving; they are constantly in giving mode. On the other hand, some people only want to receive; they are not interested in giving. The cun position gives an accurate description of a life in these terms.

How can I tell if a patient is able to fight off a common cold?
In a patient with a cold, if the cun position is floating and tight but has good width, the patient has the mediumship and the Qi to carry the pathogen out; it just needs a little help. However, it could be floating and tight but small or thin or short, in which case the patient needs more Fluids from the Middle Jiao, the Stomach. In that case, nourish Fluids. If the cun position does not float, the dispersing function of the Lungs must be restored by tonifying Wei Qi. To tonify Wei Qi one must determine where it is deficient. The Lungs may need to be released. The Stomach might be tight and need to be released so that Gu Qi can become Wei Qi. (Luo points and Shu Stream points release Ying so that it can become Wei Qi). Kidney Yang might need to be tonified because Wei Qi is a subset of Kidney Yang. The sensory orifices may be blocking the expression of Wei Qi.

How can I tell if the Cold is moving into Shao Yang or Yang Ming?
When the floating cun pulse becomes rapid, the pathogen is beginning to move into the interior into the guan position, even if you don't yet feel it in the guan position. The rapid aspect indicates that the body is developing a Yang Ming condition, generating Heat in response to the pathogen. If the cun pulse is floating and slippery, it is progressing into a Shao Yang condition. If the guan position is rapid the condition is moving into Yang Ming. If the guan position is floating, a Shao Yang condition is indicated. It does not have to be slippery or rapid because it is already inferred.

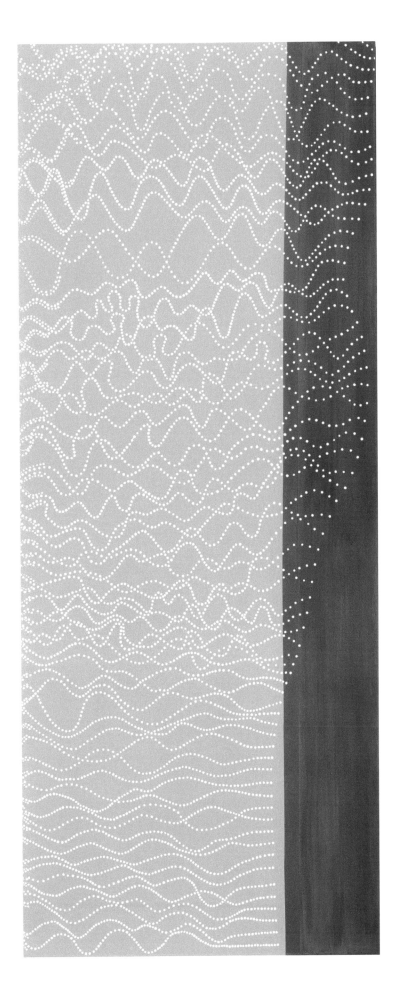

Heavenly Qi Seeps into the Bone

This work depicts the ever-present Divine force, inseparable from humankind, ever-ready to be noticed, to guide, to nurture, to reassure, to light the way. But the mind and its emotions habitually resist, pushing back on the radiance of supreme intelligence until, at last, there is an acquiescence, a yielding, a realization that the Divine is the only source of inspiration. When there is no resistance, the Divine can enter; the Blood drinks it into the pulse itself, the Divine enters the marrow, and there is wholeness.

If I am not examining vectors, how can I determine whether the Middle Jiao is supporting the Upper Jiao?

The width of the guan position pulse is what determines the level of support coming from the Middle Jiao. If the pulse is thin or small, there is limited support. If it is wide, there can be adequate support.

How can I differentiate between Fu and Zang organ pathology?

According to the *Mai Jing*, if the pulse is rapid, the Fu organ is implicated; if the pulse is slow, the Zang organ is implicated. This is because the Fu organs are Yang and move Qi whereas the Zang organs are Yin, and are more about storing Qi. A rapid pulse in the left guan position would indicate pathology of the Gallbladder.

Is a floating pulse always pathological?

A floating or dispersing pulse is only pathological at the cun if it is slow or rapid. It's pathological in any other position.

What does it mean if all the left pulses are thin?

This is a condition called visceral agitation and dryness (Zang Zao). If the left Kidney pulse is thin, there is weakness of the Kidneys and the Bladder. If the Liver pulse is thin, there may not be sufficient Blood to maintain latency, so Blood stagnation may develop. If the cun position is thin, deep and wiry it might also be weak and not communicating with the Kidney. Zang Zao results in an adversely affected Shen and in personality disorders. BL-43 is a principal point in its treatment.

What does it mean when you say that long pulses mean the organ or channel has exceeded its limits?

When the pulse has become long, it means the body has to find another way to deal with the pathogen because the pathogen cannot be contained. For example, if a floating cun position pulse becomes long and occupies the guan position as well, it means the body has exceeded its capacity to contain or expel that pathogen and transformation is taking place. The body is responding with Heat or Dampness which the Middle Jiao generates. The guan position may now be floating and slippery or floating and rapid. In the long-term, if the condition isn't resolved, the body may reach into the deep reserves of Yang Qi to mount a major fever or other healing response and the pulses will lengthen further to occupy three positions. This would be a Du Mai pulse. If Wind is prevailing, there could eventually be the risk of a stroke.

When should I be concerned that a pulse is not descending when it should?
It's essential to ensure that there is descension when you have long, floating pulse, especially a long pulse that has exceeded two positions. When there is a floating pulse involving the chi position, the body's ability to control pathology that is being held in latency is compromised.

The descending quality must be restored. Also, if there is a Triple Heater pulse, restoring the descending quality in the pulses is essential to maintaining latency of fire toxins.

I feel nothing between the top of the Wei level and the radial artery. Why?
You may feel nothing between the skin level and the artery because there is consolidation going on; the patient is anchoring resources. However, if you find the pulse pushing up as you press down beyond the artery, it means that the Yuan level is trying to release something pathological, or there is leakage occurring. If you feel something pushing back up as you release pressure but it doesn't come up to the Wei level, that is sometimes referred to as a soft pulse; it doesn't have the integrity to reach all the way back to the surface. (Although a soft pulse usually refers to a pulse that loses integrity as you press down on it.) This is a dynamic quality, not a static quality. It is only felt as you release pressure.

What aspects of the pulse should I examine in order to determine the pathology underlying a case of Blood stasis?
Deficiency of Kidney Yang and the failure of the Kidneys to communicate with the Heart are key factors in the Heart not being able to quicken Blood and break up Blood stasis. Examine the diffusing action of the Lung. Is Blood moving from the Liver to the Heart? Is there enough Liver Blood for the body to allow movement of Blood? Is there sufficient Kidney Yang to finance this movement?

Do you ever look to see whether the Kidneys are nourishing Liver Blood?
Yes. If you press down on the Kidney pulse and release from the Liver pulse, you can see whether the Kidneys are breaking down Yin to finance Blood. This vector illustrates the breaking down of Yin as an expense incurred by life. It is part of the natural process. However, it can also be indicative of the Kidneys having to expend more Blood than should be necessary because postnatal Qi is not sufficient to produce adequate Blood. In either case, if the process is not going well, the Liver will show deficiency of Blood, and nourishment of Blood is required.

When I'm deciding which Divergent Channel I can safely use, is it better to take the Divergent pulses, or to examine the mediumship available?

That's a complicated question, but in your strategy always satisfy both ways of thinking. After pressing to 15 beans, releasing slightly away from the bone to 14 beans of pressure, feeling a pulse that is beating against your finger, pushing back down to 15 beans of pressure and finding that pulse disappears, you can be confident that this particular Divergent confluence has the capacity to hold latency. This doesn't mean you should treat that Channel straight away, however. The medium this channel requires to be able to hold a pathogen in latency may be in the process of being transformed into another medium to enable a different Divergent Channel to hold latency. For example, the Heart/Small Intestine Divergent might have room (it might disappear at the second visit to 15 beans) but if Yin is being transformed into Blood so that the Gallbladder Divergent can hold latency, the Heart/Small Intestine confluence might not be the best choice. In that case the moderate level of the Liver pulse would be thin, indicating the deficit of Blood requiring that transformation from Yin resources, and the deep level of the left chi (Kidney Yin) will be thin as Yin is being sacrificed to make Blood. A vector going upward from the Kidney to the Liver will confirm that transformation. Your aim will be first to nourish Blood to take pressure off the Yin so that you can go ahead and use the Heart/Small Intestine Divergent, confident that the resources are sufficient (this could all be in one session or require more time). One could make a blanket statement, though: if the Triple Heater pulse is strong enough and you are looking for latency when a pathogen is out of control, use the Triple Heater Divergent Channel.

How can I locate Wind in the pulses?

If the pulse is floating and full, this indicates an excess condition of exterior Wind. If the pulse is superficial and tight, there is Wind trapped in the Sinews. If the pulse is rough, there is internal Wind.

What does it mean if I find a floating pulse in all three positions?

You may have found an Eight Extra pulse, likely the Du Mai pulse. On the left wrist, if you find all three positions floating from the deep level to the superficial level, something is being released from the Jing. Cup SI-12 to clear turbidity. Go back and check the pulses; they should no longer be floating. If they are, something is likely trapped in the jaw or the sensory orifices. Release SI-18 and do a Sinew treatment.

I can't find any floating pulses. What does it mean?

Gu Qi is unable to become Wei Qi. Release the Stomach. Bleed Luo points, as they bring Ying to the Wei level. Or needle Shu-Stream points, as they provide the same function.

I found rapid pulses in all three positions. What does this mean?

Chapter eight of the *Mai Jing* says that if you find the pulses rapid in all three positions during a chronic condition, the prognosis is not necessarily serious. But if the condition is acute and the pulse is rapid in all three positions, the condition is serious.

What qualities will show in the pulses if an organ is diseased?

If you find that at the deep level, the pulse is long and firm or soft and scattered, there is an issue with the Yin organ. If you find that at the moderate level the pulse is long and firm or soft and scattered, there is an issue with the Yang organ.

Why should a soft and scattered pulse indicate that the issue is in the organ?

If, as the Qi rises up it hits you in the finger and scatters, the Qi of the organ doesn't have enough integrity to extend all the way through the channels. The channels are an extension of the Zang Fu, so if the channel has surplus of Qi and Blood this surplus quality would extend into the pulses, giving you a long and firm pulse. If the organs have an insufficiency of Qi and Blood, that quality of insufficiency will extend into channels and then into the pulses as a soft and scattered quality because they lack the integrity needed to maintain the flow of Qi. The pulse then becomes soft. This indicates deficiency of the organ.

What does a long and firm pulse reflect about the pathology of an organ?

A long and firm pulse indicates an overtaxed organ due to excess in the organ. It distributes its pathology to other positions in the pulse (cun, guan or chi) and pushes back at you when you push down on it because it cannot accept any more pathology.

How can I tell if a person is able to relax or not?

If there are no tight, superficial pulses, the person is likely able to reach a relaxed state.

How can I tell if the body is hydrated?

To be fully hydrated, all the fluids need to be replete. Ying Qi supports the exterior. This is shown in the width of the moderate level. The Jin-Thin fluids moisten the skin, sinews and sensory orifices; these are shown in the Wei level of the pulse. The Ye-Thick Fluids support the bone and marrow. These are represented in the Yuan level of the pulse. We're really looking for good width throughout.

Where in the pulse can I find reflected the sense of self-worth, fulfillment and a sense of accomplishment in life?

In the width and integrity of the Ying level of the guan position. Also in the Eight Extra pulses at 15 beans of pressure.

Is a rapid pulse always pathological?

The Heart pulse is often naturally slightly rapid. Generally, though, a rapid pulse indicates Heat, either as a pathology or as a response to pathology. If the pulse is floating and rapid, the body has mounted a physiological response to Cold, opposing that pathogenic factor. A moderate and rapid pulse is pathological and over time will consume Qi, Blood and Humors. A deep and rapid pulse indicates Heat consuming Yin, resulting in an Empty Heat situation. There may be transverse cracks on the tongue in this case.

What does it mean if the pulses at the superficial level are thin?

In the cun position this shows deficient Jin-Thin Fluids. In the guan it can mean the Blood is unable to move outward to the four limbs. In the chi position, it tells you there is insufficient Yin and therefore Yang is being allowed to escape.

The Sinew treatments I am doing with a particular patient are not working. The pulse is superficial and tight, so the Sinews feel as though they are ready for release. What am I missing?

Tight superficial pulses do indicate Sinew pathology, but in order for a treatment to work, there must be sufficient Stomach Fluids, Kidney Yang, dispersing Lung Qi and unobstructed Liver Qi. Check the width of the moderate level of the right guan, the strength at the deep level of the right chi; check that the Lungs are dispersing and that the Liver pulse is not tight at any level. Treat accordingly, check the pulses again and then release the Sinews. This can all happen in the same session.

Is a tight and weak pulse deficient or excess?

Deficient. The tightness is a response to a deficiency. A pulse can be tight and weak, tight and thin, tight and empty. In these cases the tightness is not pathological because if the body wants to gather a medium, it must gather Qi. Sometimes there is desperation in the gathering and the pulse can become wiry in the long term. Thin and tight on the left guan would indicate insufficient Blood. Thin and tight on the right guan would indicate there is insufficient Jin-Ye or Stomach Yin. Thin and tight on the deep level of the chi position would indicate a deficiency of Jing-Essence. Nourish the depleted medium and the tightness will dissipate. (If the pulse were tight and full it would be an excess condition, likely of Cold.)

I understand that when the pulse is tight and also empty, weak or thin, I should nourish the medium that is depleted, but what should I do if the pulses are tight in the presence of Dampness?

In the presence of dampness, transform dampness rather than expel or drain it. This honors the body's attempt to hold on to resources.

How can I tell in the pulses if Heat is being expressed or not?

If the rapid pulse is not floating, it's not coming out.

Can we tell from the pulses where Heat will go next?

Yes. If the pulse is rapid and floating, the Heat is trying to move up and out, so it will want to move to the Upper Jiao, to the Lungs. Encourage this expression.

My patient with irregular periods has rebellious Qi and her pulses are rough. Can you comment?

If there is rebellious Qi with rough pulses, the periods may become irregular because there is a Blood deficiency together with a loss of normal rhythm. Chong Mai third and fifth trajectories would treat that.

What channels are indicated if the pulses are choppy?

Choppy pulses indicate Blood stagnation with Blood deficiency. Bleeding Luo Channels may provide the most effective treatment. Be sure to bleed HT-5 or PC-6 to treat the stagnation since these two Luos govern circulation. If the Spleen is not ascending to the Lungs, it means it is not ascending Blood from the Liver to the Heart, also. You might moxa the third trajectory of the Kidney Primary Channel by moxa-ing KI-2 and SP-8 to ascend the Spleen.

My patient's pulses were thin so I am nourishing Yin but now the pulses are becoming slippery instead of wider. What am I doing wrong?

Thin pulses may mean that there is a deficiency of Yin but there could be a Yin deficiency because the body is unable to store Yin. If the Kidneys cannot store Yin and you work to nourish Yin, you can create Yin pathology (Dampness). Sometimes that Dampness can slow down the Yin leading to Wind-Phlegm. The condition is being made worse. The Heart provides the Qi for consolidation as it moves down to the Kidneys. Communicate the Heart down to the Kidneys to enable the body to store Yin.

Why do the pulses of the Yin Sinews show up in the superficial level, rather than in the deep level?

When examining the presence of pathology in the Sinews, the Yang stages reflect Wei Qi fighting the pathology off, while the Yin stages reflect the depletion of Wei Qi. Since the Sinews are the conduits of Wei Qi, all pathology of the Sinew Channels must show up in the Wei level.

How can I determine the prognosis of the disease from the pulses?

The Spirit is what determines the prognosis. Examine the pulse at the left cun. If it is dispersing to the superficial level, prognosis is better than if not. Pulse-taking is not just a technical evaluation but part of the process of cultivating awareness of the way the patient sees the world. One of the gifts of pulse-taking is that through taking the pulse we can transmit the feeling that all is well, no matter what. We can transmit the feeling that Destiny is playing out and that the Will can steer it. Touch is far more powerful than talking. When we are born, we yearn for touch rather than sound. Touch provides the ultimate comfort; pulse-taking is an opportunity to be in that beautiful and basic human space.

How do I know what kinds of questions to ask, given my observations about the pulse in the three levels?

If you were examining the left cun pulse, for example, and you found the pulse at the superficial level floating and tight, ask about the Sinews related to that area: the scapulae, shoulders and elbows. If there are pathological qualities at the moderate level, ask about the bowels, urination (since the Small Intestine passes its pathology to its zonal pair, the Bladder), or the Heart Channel. If you found pathological qualities in the deep level, ask about the Heart organ itself.

How can I tell where in the body an issue with a given Sinew Channel is located?

If the Sinew pulse is floating and slippery, think low in the body since Dampness is heavy. If the Sinew pulse is floating and rapid, think high because Heat rises. If a Sinew pulse has become rapid, ask about the next most Yang region since the body is trying to vent the pathology further to the exterior. For example, a rapid Shao Yang Sinew pulse may be expressing in Tai Yang as the channel moves the pathology out to the exterior.

Why is it said that Sinew pulses on the left wrist are more serious than those found on the right wrist?

The left Sinew pulses show more severe conditions because the left pulses reflect the body's capacity for latency. If the body is unable to produce latency (if it is unable to hide the pathogen away relatively safely, given its inability to eradicate it) sinew pulses may show on the left as the pathology seeps out. By this stage, the pathology has become severe.

I found an Eight Extra pulse, and while I was treating the Channel, that pulse disappeared. What happened?

The body felt that it was returning to balance.

Are Eight Extra pulses always pathological?

Not always. For example, a Yin Wei Mai pulse might appear if the patient is experiencing a hormonal shift or a life transition. That would not be pathological. It just means that Yin

216

Wei Mai is acting to assimilate the playing out of Destiny.

Why are Eight Extra pulses moving pulses?

The vibrating quality reflects an uneasiness either with change, with who we are, with being in our own skin, with our environment. Or it can vibrate because we are being prevented from being who we are. Perhaps there has been trauma and there is Fright-Wind (post-traumatic stress) causing a lack of ease in the present moment. Chronic trauma or abuse by parents or a spouse may have undermined the patient's ability to feel comfortable in him/herself. They reactively want to alter their Jing-Essence. The patient rations their Jing differently. But Jing is supposed to be consistent; it keeps oneself in the present, in reality and keeps the form intact. If the Mind is calm, the Jing will be calm, not moving.

What is implied if I cannot get the pulses to change in my dialogue with the pulse?

If you cannot change the pulse by suggesting that it change using your intention while taking the pulse, there is most likely a visceral (organ) problem. Substance changes more slowly than energy. If the pulse is rapid and doesn't want to change, most likely you are finding inflammation of the organ itself. If it is the channels that are affected, acupuncture will have a greater and more immediate effect. If the pathology is of the organ, acupuncture will be effective, but take longer.

Is it possible to feel the antique points indicated in the pulses?

The Jing-Well is felt at the superficial level, the Shu-Stream at the moderate level and the He-Sea at the deep level. If the pulses are rapid, the Ying-Spring points are indicated. If slow, the Jing-River points. If the pulses are tight, the Xi-Cleft point is indicated. If the pulse is choppy, the Luo points are appropriate. This approach could be the foundation of another book on pulses.

Is it possible to determine the indication of the Source, Mu or Shu points?

The pulses do not have point categories, but if you wanted to practice that way and the pulses are weak, you might tonify the Bladder Shu points or the Yin Source points. If they are slippery, you might reduce them. If the pulses are full, you might work with the Mu points, as Mu points work with excesses, or reduce the Yang Source points.

How should I treat a knotted pulse?

The knotted pulse indicates stagnation of Yin. Nourish Yin so that it can move. If you're interested in the roots and terminations, the Yin Channels terminate in the throat, chest and abdomen. SP-1 terminates at CV-12. LR-1 terminates at CV-18 then CV-17. KI-1 terminates at CV-22 and CV-23. When there is stagnation of Yin, these are areas of distress. If the pulses are also tight, needle the Xi-Cleft points first, then clear Heat or scatter Cold.

What are the psychological aspects of tight or wiry pulses?

Since tight or wiry pulses show stagnation, they reflect the inability to let go. There may be hoarding pathology, living in clutter, inability to throw things out. There may be a tendency for the patient to settle for that which is not best for them or to accumulate what is not necessary, compensating for underlying deficiencies, whether physical, energetic or mental. There is likely difficulty relaxing, being at ease. The patient may be clutching at aspects of life.

Is it always the case that if there is an excess somewhere in the pulses, there will be a deficiency elsewhere in the pulses?

Yes. A slippery pulse in the Lung position, for instance, may be indicating Dampness, but on a deeper level it may be indicating that the Lung is unable to diffuse Qi. Perhaps there is an underlying Yin deficiency or Kidney Yang deficiency.

Is it possible to tell whether a disease is fatal?

It's important for the practitioner to keep focusing on the patient's health, rather than the disease. A crucial part of the clinical process is to focus on all the good that can come to and from a patient's life. To be effective, the practitioner must focus on the best the patient can be. Focus on healing; imagine the patient is healed. They will determine what healing is, and embody the treatment as fits their Destiny.

How would I see insomnia in the pulses?

Any condition in any person is a unique combination of many factors. These factors differ from patient to patient. There is no textbook pulse presentation of any condition. Every set of signs and symptoms will show differently in every person's pulses. That is why it is essential to take pulses and then provide the treatment that is uniquely appropriate for that patient.

Is there a pulse that best reflects how a patient is doing on that day?

The cun position reflects what the patient is experiencing in the immediate term. Common colds will show up in the cun, not the chi, for example. Enthusiasm about the day itself shows in the cun. Heat generated in that morning's gym session will show up in the cun.

Do the pulse positions reflect anatomical areas?

Yes, the chi position represents the body inferior to Dai Mai. The guan position reflects the area between Dai Mai and the diaphragm, and the cun position represents the body superior to the diaphragm.

Which is the most important pulse?

That depends on your style of practice. Analysis of the Lung pulse is historically very significant. The release of the exterior that is dependent on the Lungs is the focus of the *Shang Han Lun* tradition. That tradition is founded upon expelling a Tai Yang condition to prevent transmission to a deeper level. But Lung Qi is derived from the Middle Jiao, so the guan position is very important; postnatal Qi is determined by digestive health. And of course, the chi position represents the foundation of all Yin and Yang. They are all equally important.

How does immunity show in the pulse?

If the Lungs are strong at the Wei level and the Stomach pulse is wide at the moderate level, there is enough defensive Qi and enough Fluids to defend the exterior. To demonstrate good immunity, both pulses should push back slightly. Wang Shu He says that Yang is engendered in the chi position and manifests in the cun, causing the cun to float, and Yin is engendered at the cun position and manifests in the chi position, causing the chi to be deep. If this cycle is evident in the pulses, immunity can be sound.

Where would I look for memory loss in the pulses?

As you push into the moderate level of the Liver pulse, it should give way to the Jing level. It should be quite wide. If it's thin, there's a decline in the marrow or the bone. This may result in memory loss, since the Marrow is the sum total of Jing-Essence and Shen. Marrow enables the recall of time.

What does it mean if the pulses are superficial, rapid and slippery all at the same time?

The exterior is blocked and the ability to release is compromised. Pathology must have an outlet. A blocked exterior is like having sealed-off exits.

All the left pulse positions: the Heart, Liver and Kidneys float from the deep level to about three beans.

Something has been released from the Jing and is trapped. Cup SI-12 which clears turbidity. After cupping the pulse should give way. If it doesn't, there's probably something trapped in the jaw or the sensory orifices which is more serious. Needle to release SI-18 before continuing with the treatment you decide on.

I feel nothing at all in any position until I reach the radial artery at nine beans.

This means there is consolidation occurring. The body is in conservation mode reserving mediumship.

What should I do if I find the pulses floating and superficial in all three positions?

When this happens, always check to see if they are moving. Moving pulses call you to examine the Eight Extra pulses, then the Divergent pulses.

QUESTIONS ABOUT THE CUN POSITION

What can I do if the pulse at the cun position is consistently absent?
Try treating it as a physiological blockage. Do a sinew treatment that includes the torso to stimulate Wei Qi so the pulse can go all the way up to the cun position and out.

What are the implications of a thin cun pulse on the left side?
A thin pulse in the superficial level of the left cun position indicates a deficiency in the Small Intestine which may result in a hormonal deficiency because the Small Intestine controls the Ye-Thick Fluids. If the moderate level of the cun position is thin, Liver Blood is not nourishing Heart Blood.

When is a floating pulse pathological at the cun?
A floating pulse is only pathological at the cun position if it is slow or rapid.

Why can I not find a floating pulse in the cun position?
Either there is no support from the Ying level or there's no support from the Yuan level. Ying Qi or Yang Qi is not supporting Wei Qi. Or, there is a blockage of the sensory orifices. These blockages can lead to allergies, sinus discharge, eye discharge, all indicating the orifices are blocked. The diaphragm might also be blocked.

No matter what I do, I can't get the Lung pulse to stop being thin.
Examine the Stomach pulse. Fluids are likely not being conveyed to the Lungs. If the Stomach pulse is tight or wiry, Fluids from the Middle Jiao cannot reach the Upper Jiao. Release the Stomach by nourishing Fluids. Also, check to see that the Spleen is ascending Fluids from the Middle Jiao to the Lungs.

What does it mean if the Lung pulse scatters at the moderate level?
Qi, Yin or Fluids are coming up to the cun position but are being used up too quickly. This is called Dryness of the Blood or Dryness of the Yin.

I can't get Lung Qi to descend. What does it mean?
This means Yang Qi cannot be anchored. Wind signs and symptoms such as seizures and convulsions can result. Ask about low back issues. A tight low back means the Kidneys are likely tight and unable to receive Qi or Yin from the Lungs. If you release the low back, the Lungs might descend straight away. Blockages in the diaphragm can block descension, also.

What does it mean if the Lung pulse is soft?
If you press the Lung pulse down to three beans and find it floating and tight and then add

a little more pressure, taking it to between four and six beans and finding nothing there, the pulse is said to be soft. That tells you that the body hasn't the resources to push out a pathogenic factor. Press deeper to see where the pathogenic factor has gone. Where has the body put it? This is revealed when the pulse becomes tight or rapid or slippery. It has to go to the ditches, the Luo points or the Source points. If the pulse is rough it may go to the Blood level because there's not enough blood to resist it.

What does it mean if despite really trying to do qigong on the Lung pulse, it will not disperse?
The Lung pulse should float. Everyone should have floating pulses at the cun level. Everyone should be expressing their Qi and Blood. Life is being expressed and there's no embarrassment, shyness or holding back. If there is no floating pulse in the cun, you should be able to create one by pressing the guan and releasing from the cun as described in chapter 3. If you cant't, the patient is unable to adapt to change, or there's a blockage between the guan and cun positions.

I'm trying to get the Lungs to diffuse Qi but I'm not having any success. The Spleen ascends to the Lungs. What am I missing?
The Lung pulse may be unable to diffuse Qi because the Lungs are obstructed by Dampness. The Spleen to Lungs vector may be present (the Spleen may be ascending its Qi to the Lungs as desired) but during that ascension, the Dampness is moving with the Qi, and being deposited in the Lungs. This is weighing down the Lungs, making them unable to diffuse.

Or, perhaps the Lungs are Yin deficient and they are reactively retaining that Dampness. Yin stasis often develops due to an underlying Yin deficiency. The Dampness is preventing the Lungs dispersing. Nourishing Yin will allow the Dampness to be expelled. Or, perhaps the patient just lost a family member or a job and is suppressing grief by retaining Dampness in the Lungs. Bleeding the Luo Channels will move Blood to move the emotions, releasing the emotional pressure on the Lungs.

My patient's Lung pulse is beady and I can't seem to open the Lungs up. The Spleen is ascending. There's plenty of Kidney Yang and the Liver is not tight.
The Lungs are the center of guilt, grief, redemption, justice, fairness, forgiveness and acceptance. The beadiness (accumulation) may be reflecting your patient's inability to let go of something. Stasis in the Lungs may be due to unfulfilled desires or an underlying deficiency. The treatment principle, then, is to nourish the deficiency rather than to unblock the accumulation. Nourish Yin. Just a thought: You don't mention the Heart in your question. Examine the Eight Extra pulses and see if there's a Yin Wei Mai pulse there.

My patient's Lungs will not diffuse or descend. The Lung pulse is thin and rapid.
The Lungs will not diffuse and descend if the Lung pulse is rapid, slow, slippery, thin or wiry. If the pulse is thin, it's important to nourish fluids. Then use the points you learned in school that descend and disperse the Lungs. (LU-7 does both, of course. LU-8 allows the Lungs to let go.)

What makes the Lung pulse thin?
Often this is due to tightness in the Stomach, restricting its ability to share nourishment with the Lungs. A thin cun pulse reveals a problem with the guan position.

I understand that tight pulses very often indicate that the body is trying to conserve a medium, but I found a tight pulse in the Large Intestine. What could this mean?
Sometimes tight simply means Cold is present. Ask about undigested food in the stools, constipation or cramping. Use moxa. The Large Intestine controls the Jin-Thin Fluids; perhaps there's a deficiency there.

If I want to see whether the Large Intestine is performing its function of managing Jin-Thin fluids, what level of the pulse should I look at?
When analyzing the Large Intestine you're interested in the width at the moderate level of the right cun where it's function of management of Jin-Thin Fluids is evident. That tells you whether or not it is capable of managing Fluids. The Wei level will tell you how much Jin-Thin fluid is being produced.

What might a long and firm right cun pulse indicate?
Lung organ issues such as wheezing, coughing and difficulty breathing.

No matter how much I try to tonify Lung Qi, I cannot get the Lungs to float. (Yes, the Spleen is ascending to the Lungs.)
Some people will not have or develop floating pulses because they don't really want to engage with the world. That might be an aspect of their nature.

What is indicated when the right cun pulse is very tight at the deep level?
The Lungs are likely trying to move Cold out through the Lower Jiao since the Upper Jiao failed to expel the Cold. This patient probably has very frequent urination as the Lower Jiao tries to drain the pathology.

What happens if the Lungs and Stomach are not descending?
The Lungs and Stomach are not nourishing Kidney Qi. The Lungs and the Stomach are the postnatal Qi receptors and both must descend to support Kidney Qi. It is important to

determine which of the two organs is not descending and then to treat that channel.

Some books say the Pericardium is in the left cun position. Why?
The Pericardium became identified with the left cun during the Song Dynasty, a theoretical shift that has been widely accepted.

What might a long and firm left cun pulse indicate?
This could be the Hidden Beam pulse. The Hidden Beam is a tightness in Chong Mai sometimes known as chopstick Qi.

Why might the Heart pulse push back at my finger as I press into the moderate level?
As you push down on the cun position, it should give with the pressure. If the pulse gets stronger as you move to the more moderate level, it indicates that there is a reluctance to rest; the patient is overextending him/herself.

You're talking about the left pulses giving way to pressure indicating they can deal with pathology if need be, and at the same time, you say the Heart pulse should scatter. How can both be happening at the same time?
The Heart pulse should only give way upon increased pressure from your finger. When you're taking the Heart pulse and you release pressure from it, in the absence of pathology, it will scatter, disperse or float. This upward movement is a desired quality. On a philosophical level, the floating pulse represents the meeting of the Heart and the Qi of heaven, the mandate from Heaven. The yielding of the Heart pulse represents the acceptance of heavenly Qi. If we are able to meet and accept the Qi of Heaven and its light, we are able to know with certainty what it is we are here to do.

I feel the Heart descending Qi but I don't feel the Kidneys grasping it. Why?
There's not enough Yin to anchor down the Yang from the Heart. Or, the body does not have the capacity to store that Yin. If it can't store Yin, the Yin that you build in treatments does not have a place to be; it's not consolidated. The Yin that you build in treatments, if not consolidated, can move around the body, as Wind-Phlegm. The condition can become chronic. The Qi of consolidation comes from the Heart. Communicate the Heart downward. KI-21 has this function, as does Bao Mai.

What does it mean if the Heart pulse is rapid?
A rapid Heart pulse may mean that Heat issues relating to the Heart are being moved to the elemental pair, the Small Intestine. From there, the body can pass the pathology to the Small Intestine's zonal pair, the Bladder.

What does it mean if there is a beady pulse in the Heart position?

This often occurs with severe trauma or major life disappointments. It indicates Blood stagnation or significantly suppressed anger.

What should I find at the deep level of the Heart pulse?

When you go deep in the Heart pulse it should feel stable and balanced. If it feels full, there is Pericardium activity; Blood is being held back. If so, calm the Shen.

Is it normal for the Heart pulse to be slightly rapid?

Yes, the Heart pulse can be slightly rapid without it being pathological. This is common in people of great enthusiasm, with a zest for life.

I found a rough, rapid, very strong, pounding, full pulse in the deep level of the left cun. What does it mean?

You are describing an urgent pulse. This is not to be confused with flooding. A flooding pulse is found on the superficial level. An urgent pulse feels like a flooding pulse but it's found on the deep level. This indicates a functional problem in the Heart. It could be valvular, mitral valve prolapse or cardiac regurgitation. It could be entitic.

What does it mean if instead of feeling a vector going from the Liver to the Heart, I feel a vector going from the Heart to the Liver?

This would mean that there has not been enough sleep and the Heart is trying to send Blood back to the Liver to induce the sleep state.

What does it mean if the Heart pulse becomes long as I press down into the moderate level?

If any pulse becomes long, it means that the organ is not able to cope with the sum of its pathology. It is trying to share the burden. If the left cun position pulse becomes long as you press into the moderate level, that is, if it extends to include the Gallbladder, there may be Gallbladder organ issues or Small Intestine organ issues.

What is the significance of a thin pulse in the Wei level of the Heart pulse?

The Wei level of the Heart pulse should scatter as you release or soften as you press down on it a little within the Wei level. A thin pulse in the Wei level of this position indicates a possible hormonal deficiency because the Small Intestine controls the Ye-Thick Fluids and the Thick Fluids are not anchored.

If I don't want to look at a person's spiritual orientation, why should I examine the pulses to see if the Heart and the Kidneys communicate?

This vector is a marker of strength. If the Heart and Kidneys communicate, there is sufficient strength to allow the Heart to regulate or create evenness in the pulses. It is the circulation of the microcosmic orbit that allows processes in the body to be rhythmic. Hasty, knotted, intermittent, irregular pulses that occlude this communication indicate pathology; something is preventing the circuitry from being open and free to communicate. This is every bit as physical as it is spiritual.

What does it mean if the Heart pulse is rapid and strongly floating?

It means Heat is moving up to the head to vent. If the Lung pulse is behaving the same way, there are likely headaches with menstruation. If the Heart pulse is rapid and moderate, Heat is going to the Bladder via the Small Intestine, causing urinary tract infections. If it is deep, it means it is going to the Kidneys and damaging Jing-Essence. This can occur in situations of deep emotional stress, or even at postpartum.

I can't get the Heart pulse to widen despite many treatments.

All Heart Blood and Heart Qi originates in Liver Blood. Nourish Liver Blood. The Heart pulse will widen immediately.

QUESTIONS ABOUT THE GUAN POSITION

Why would the guan position pulse float?

This could indicate a Sinew condition (Wind trapped in the Sinews) or there are insufficient Fluids or Blood to contain Qi, allowing Qi to float. Heat in the Stomach or the Gallbladder can also cause the pulse to float.

Can the guan position float because it is supporting the cun position?

Yes. Wei Qi is a product of Da Qi supported by Gu Qi. Wei Qi comes from the turbid fluids; the Yin of the Gu. Therefore during a healing episode, when Ying is transforming into Wei Qi, the guan level can float because it's supporting that level.

What are the reasons the guan position might be consistently tight?

1. Diaphragm blockage.
2. There might be insufficient Yang Qi to reach the head. (If indicated, release GV-14 where all Yang channels meet.)
3. If it's tight at the superficial level, Bi-Obstruction may be affecting the four limbs. The body is trying to release something from the Middle Jiao but it can't because the four limbs are blocking it. If the guan is floating, the cun should be also, because what the body wants to release can be brought to the exterior. If the guan is floating and cun is not, there

is a blockage. This is very common. It may obstruct treatments if it is not treated first.

4. Deficiency of Blood or Fluids. The Middle Jiao is trying to gather or conserve fluids and becomes tight as it does so.

What does it mean if I only find a pulse in the guan position?

It could mean that the body is unable to make enough Qi, Blood and Fluids to distribute, so nothing is being expressed or stored.

Is it a bad sign if the guan is floating?

If the guan AND the cun are floating, that's not bad; things are coming out. If the guan is floating but the cun is not, there is a blockage.

There are no pulses at the Wei level. The Stomach pulse is tight. What should I do?

Gu Qi is unable to become Wei Qi. Release the Stomach by tonifying what is lacking. Then bleed the Luo points because they are responsible for bringing Ying to the Wei level. Shu-Stream points also perform this action.

What should I look for if the Spleen is not ascending?

Look for impedance to the movement of Spleen Qi. The most common of these is Dampness, so look for slipperiness in the Spleen. If the Spleen pulse is wiry, it certainly cannot ascend. If you can't find anything in the static pulses, check the vectors between organs by examining the directional pulses. The impedance might be coming from somewhere other than the Spleen. If the Heart is tight, that may affect the Spleen because the Spleen Primary Channel has an internal branch that goes to the Heart. Tightness in the Liver can also affect its neighbor, the Spleen.

I very often find the Spleen is slightly slippery. Is this okay?

It depends on the level and the time. When the Spleen is active in digestion the Spleen can be slightly slippery on the moderate level because to digest food, as in cooking, you must have the right balance of fluids. It's not okay for the Spleen to be slippery on the deep level. This would indicate pathology affecting the organ itself. It should not be slippery at any level when there are other qualities present at that level such as tight and scattered.

I cannot get the Stomach to descend despite regular treatment.

The patient is doing something on a regular basis to cause the Stomach to be in constant rebellion. This is often food related. Cold or frozen food and drinks are among the most common factors, but there are many.

What might it mean if I find a deviated pulse in the Spleen position?

Deviated pulses are those in which all three pulses can be felt in an alternative set of positions, or a single pulse can be felt in an additional location. They can indicate the patient has double the strength. If you feel the Spleen in two positions for the Spleen, the Qi of the Spleen is plentiful.

I found a rapid pulse in the Yuan level of the Spleen position. What does it mean?

It means that Heat in Yang Ming (the Stomach) is affecting the elementally paired organ. If not treated, Wei Atrophy Syndrome (neuropathy) may result from depletion of Fluids in the Middle Jiao. If the Spleen pulse is also slippery, disinhibit the Dampness.

As I press from the superficial level into the moderate level of the Spleen pulse, it gets stronger, indicating descension of the Stomach, but as I continue to press into the deep level, the pulse tightens. What does this mean both physically and mentally?

This means Qi and Blood are not regulated. The patient is unable to muster discipline, to allocate time to their various responsibilities.

There's a very full and pronounced pulse at the deep level of the right guan position. What does this mean?

The patient has been unable to set clear and firm boundaries in the world and is experiencing limits to their tolerance of it. They uncomplainingly take on too many things. They are Damp like a sponge, soaking things in and allowing them to permeate. These patients can develop fire toxins in the Jing.

Why might the Stomach pulse be tight or wiry?

Any tight or wiry quality in the guan can be indicative of Qi, Blood or Phlegm stagnation. Often the cause is weakness of the Spleen. Press down further, into the deep level, and see whether the pulse becomes much weaker. If so, the Stomach is tight because the Spleen is unable to transform and transport. These situations arise because, due to lack of Will, there is too much rich food, addictions, or too many things accumulated. The Kidneys are therefore not supporting the Spleen. If the Spleen is truly deficient, the Stomach will become deficient, also. If there is an excess in the Stomach, first harmonize the Stomach and Spleen. There are many points that do this. I love to use SP-4 for this purpose, although ST-37, ST-40 and ST-42, of course, all perform that function.

Why do I often find that the right guan is the widest pulse?

Yang Ming has the greatest amount of Qi and Blood. This is normal. Shao Yang is less Yang so the left guan dilates less.

On the right wrist, my patient has a rapid pulses in the cun and guan positions but only at the moderate level. What might this mean?

The Lungs are trying to vent something from the Middle Jiao. Be sure to vent the Heat in the Lungs to the superficial level.

What might a long and firm pulse in the moderate level of the right guan indicate?

On the right at the moderate level, the pulse might indicate slowness of the digestive tract, food stasis, food stagnation or loss of appetite.

What might a long and firm right guan pulse at the deep level indicate?

This is indicative of edema, overflowing pathological Fluids or Phlegm. The turbidity can overflow into the four limbs, then seep out, forming limbic edema. When the pulse is like this, pathological fluids have stretched the capacity of the Spleen to handle Damp; it doesn't have enough Qi to transform the turbidity and accumulation results. There could be borborygmus and focal distention. Pulses become long and firm when excesses are in play. They become short, soft and scattered with deficiencies.

I found wiry pulses in the Liver. Does that mean there is Blood stagnation?

Wiry pulses in the Liver, Spleen or Heart do not necessarily signify true Blood stagnation. A wiry pulse may actually be indicating a long-term underlying deficiency. When the pulse has become wiry, the effort to conserve has been going on so long the Blood itself is stagnating.

What does it mean if the Gallbladder pulse is thin?

The Gallbladder controls the Marrow. As you reach the moderate level of the pulse, there should be good width. It should feel cushiony and allow you to move toward the bone with no resistance. If it is thin, it means that there is a decline in Marrow or the bone; memory cannot be retained.

If it's good for the Liver pulse to be slightly tight, is it even better when it's wiry?

It should not be wiry; that would mean it's working too hard to store Blood. Emotional issues may ensue.

The patients I see in the evening hours generally have tighter Liver pulses than those I see during the day. Why?

This is natural. In the evening, Blood is being moved back to the Liver to be stored in preparation for sleep.

Should the Liver pulse be particularly tight after menses?

Yes, the Liver pulse should be slightly tight at all times, but a little tighter after the completion of the period as Blood is stored again. If much blood was lost, it could be wiry. If there is urgency to regain Blood, the pulse could become rapid in the short term.

Why does coffee make the pulses wiry?

The coffee bean (seed) has a Liver affinity and is bitter and astringent. Even without caffeine (more with), coffee stimulates and tightens the Liver and Gall Bladder. As it is also dehydrating, the Liver must hold back Blood due to systemic dehydration. Over time, this leads to stagnation of the Liver (and a reactive addiction to coffee).

Why do Liver pulses become choppy?

The Liver is likely trying to store Blood that is not there.

Why would the Liver pulse be thin when there is plenty of sleep and excellent nourishment in the diet?

The Liver sends Blood to the Kidneys for their nourishment. If there are issues related to self-esteem, the Kidneys may be draining the resources of the Liver. Self-esteem is only possible when there is a good compliment of Kidney Yin.

What does it mean if the Liver pulse is slippery?

It means the Liver is not harmonized with the Stomach and Spleen. Harmonize the Spleen and Stomach and then harmonize the Middle Jiao.

What are the psychological factors involved in a wiry Liver pulse?

The Liver pulse can become wiry to block the Blood from being able to nourish the Kidneys and the Heart. In preventing nourishment of the Kidneys, the patient is relieved from having to examine issues related to his/her sense of self-worth. Blockage of Blood to the Heart blocks one's enthusiasm and relieves the patient from having to engage in activities of self-fulfillment. This combination occurs when there is overwhelming doubt about what one is capable of. Treat by warming the Gallbladder to conquer fear.

Why can't I generate a vector from the Liver to the Heart?

The Liver might not be able to engender Heart Blood for a variety of reasons. If the Liver pulse is slippery, there is likely Blood stasis. Bleeding the Luo Channels is particularly useful in these cases. If the pulse is wiry, the vector might not appear. If the diaphragm is blocked, Liver Blood will not be able to cross into the Upper Jiao.

Why is the Liver pulse tighter in the early Spring?

In early Spring, the earth is beginning to loosen up so that Wood can penetrate through the earth and sprout. There is a certain hesitation, tightness, or wiry quality. The pulses are still tight and not ready to fully release. When you push down, you still feel some resistance. You might even feel that when you push down further, it becomes leathery.

What does it mean if the Liver pulse is very deep?

This often means that the Gallbladder is sending resources to the brain and Marrow. It could also mean that Blood is financing habituation, for example, addiction.

What does it mean when the Liver pulse is thin at the moderate level and when you press down on it, the same thinness is felt at the moderate level of the Heart position?

It means that Liver Blood is deficient and is having trouble financing Heart Blood.

What does it mean if the Liver pulse scatters?

The Liver is not storing Blood.

What does it mean if the Gallbladder pulse is floating?

The body is trying to free something from the Gallbladder. There could be gallstones or abscesses.

If I find a long or soft pulse in the Liver position. Does that mean the Liver organ is affected?

The organ is affected if the pulse is soft and scattered, or long and firm. It is the dual nature of the qualities that indicates organ pathology. If you find a long pulse but you don't find resistance, it's simply a long but not firm pulse. That would not mean the pathology is in the organ.

What might a long and firm pulse at the moderate level of the left guan indicate?

It might indicate fatty Qi (nodules in the abdomen only palpable when the patient is lying down). There may be a bitter taste, flank distention, sour reflux and nausea as the Gallbladder cannot bring enough Qi to assist in digestion.

What might a long and firm pulse at the deep level of the left guan indicate?

There might be lateral costal pain, food stagnation, issues related to the genitalia, sterility, impotence, testicular pain and dragging pain in the low back.

What does it mean if the Liver pulse becomes tight as I am talking about childhood trauma?

If the guan pulse gets tight while you're talking about suppression at the Yuan level, then a lot of Blood has been occupied keeping those memories buried.

The Liver and Heart pulses are both thin at about 12 beans of pressure in my patient who has Multiple Sclerosis. What medium should I nourish?
This indicates that the media under the command of the Gallbladder and of the Small Intestine are deficient: Marrow and Ye-Thick Fluids, respectively.

QUESTIONS ABOUT THE CHI POSITION

The Kidney pulse is supposed to be deep and consolidating. What does it mean if it's floating to the Wei level?
If the chi position pulse floats to the Wei level, Yang Qi is escaping. There might be respiratory or dermatological conditions. Wind may be occupying the Blood causing dizziness.

What does it mean if the Bladder pulse is thin?
The Bladder controls the Sinews. If the Bladder pulse is thin, it means the scene is set for Wei Atrophy Syndrome (neuropathy) because the lack of moisture prevents maintenance of the tonicity of the sinews. There must be enough Yin to maintain the integrity of the structure and to deal with pathogenic factors.

I have been working on draining Damp and discover that a Bladder pulse has emerged at the moderate level of the left chi position. Is this to be expected?
Yes.

Is it normal for the Kidney pulse to be slightly slow?
Yes. The Kidney pulse reflects the status of Jing, which has a heavy, dense nature.

Why is the Kidney pulse referred to as the "stone pulse"?
Qi moves from the Spleen into the right Kidney via Triple Heater. The Qi is drawn into the deep level to conserve and consolidate. The Kidney pulse, therefore, is healthy when it is quiet, heavy, stone-like.

What does it mean if the Kidney Yang pulse is floating and tight?
If the Kidney Yang pulse is floating and tight it means the body is trying to prevent leakage of some kind. Zong Qi (gathering Qi) can be tight as it tries to anchor Qi. As you press down on the pulse, note whether it becomes stronger. It should become fuller, more present. If it doesn't, it means there is insufficient Yin to hold the Yang Qi down. Or, it means the Stomach and Lungs are not helping to descend Qi back down to the Kidneys. You would ascertain whether that is

the case by consulting the cun position and the vectors between the Lungs and Kidneys and the Stomach and Kidneys. If the Lungs are not descending to the Kidneys, KI-26 is indicated. If the Stomach is not descending to the Kidneys, KI-23 is indicated. These points provide anchoring.

I'm confused about how many organs are represented in the right chi position.

There are three: Kidney Yang, Triple Heater and Pericardium. Pericardium will show up at the moderate level of the right chi—which otherwise is free of pulses—if the Pericardium is blocking communication between the Heart and Kidneys. This creates stagnation in the Lower Jiao leading to Blood stasis conditions such as endometriosis and fibroids, especially if the Pericardium pulse is wiry. Nourish Blood, warm the Lower Jiao and create communication between the Heart and Kidneys using Da Bao and Bao Mai, perhaps. If the Kidney pulse is very slow, there is Cold in the Lower Jiao.

I am finding many teenagers and very young adults (particularly women) with floating pulses at the right chi. Why?

Currently, the teenage and early adult population is overstimulated by electronic screens and they are not going to bed before 10pm or 11pm. Even the idea of that sounds ridiculous to them as a group. Consequently, they are not able to produce sufficient Blood and Yin. Menstruation and fertility are becoming deeply affected. Anemia is becoming commonplace. In this population, it's common to find the right chi floating as Kidney Yang moves up to the chest to lend Yang to stimulate the production of Blood. This is not to be confused with a Triple Heater pulse.

My patient has genital itch and I found the Kidneys weak and rapid and unable to grasp Lung Qi. What could be the scenario there?

If the Kidneys cannot grasp Lung Qi, Yang escapes because it is not anchored. This manifests as Heat and Wind (itch). If there is Dampness in the Middle Jiao, instead of rising to escape and manifesting as hypertension or headaches, the Heat and Wind can be blocked by the Dampness and can only go down. Yang then manifests in the lower region with rapid pulses. But there are many possibilities.

Where would a blockage in the Bladder organ show up?

Urinary blockages show up at between six and nine beans of pressure because the Bladder is trying to let something go. It could be long and firm, or even short if there is a blockage because there is not enough Qi to move it out. As a result there is some type of urinary obstruction.

What signs and symptoms might one see if the left chi pulse at the deep level is soft and scattered?

There may be low back pain, infertility, impotence—issues related to depleted Jing-Essence.

What signs and symptoms might one see if the right chi pulse at the deep level is soft and scattered?

Triple Heater is failing to control Qi. There may be edema, swellings or leakage.

What signs and symptoms might one see if the right chi pulse at the moderate level is soft and scattered or long and firm?

This is a type of Pericardium pulse. It is reflecting a Heart condition, either physical or psychological, for example, Running Piglet Qi. Classically the Pericardium is in the moderate level of the right chi position.

My cancer patient's Liver is not nourishing Kidney Yin. Does this have an impact on his ability to generate latency of the pathogen? His pulses are all frail, especially in the chi positions.

Yes. Normally, the Liver prioritizes to the Heart, to engender Heart Qi and Blood. If the body is trying to create latency, it's imperative the Liver communicate in both directions. It may even be found prioritizing to the Kidneys. Since these deep diseases often have the emotions as a primary cause, the absence of the vector from Liver to Heart is in keeping with the desire of the patient to continue not to examine his/her emotions or do the work of healing and releasing them.

In a situation where latency is required, the Liver must descend to the Kidneys to help consolidate Yin so that a pathogenic factor can be brought into latency. Your intention would be to get the Liver to bring Blood to the Kidneys to hold the Qi since the pulses are frail (Qi and Yang are weak). The Triple Heater Divergent treatment would help the body recognize it is dealing with something toxic. The Liver can then bring its Blood to the Kidneys.

In directional pulse practice, how can I discern the difference between the ascension of the Spleen and whether the Kidneys are able to assist the Lungs in dispersing Qi?

To check thoroughly whether the Lungs' dispersing function is being generated by the Kidneys, go to Pulse Neutral position, add a little pressure to the chi position, release a tiny amount of pressure from the guan position and then quickly release a little pressure from the cun position. If you do this quickly enough, you will feel a surge of Qi coming up from the chi to the cun if Kidney Yang is financing Wei Qi. It takes practice. The ascension of the Spleen is the second leg of that action (between the guan and the cun positions).

If I want to determine whether the Kidneys are grasping Lung Qi, do I have to see if the Lungs are descending?

The Kidneys are not able to grasp Qi if the Lungs are not descending. Measure the two actions together. Press on the Lung pulse and release the Kidneys. If that mechanism is operating, the Lungs will be felt to descend and you will feel the Kidney pulse reacting as it receives that Qi.

Can Lung Qi be descending but Kidneys failing to grasp that Qi? How does that show in the pulses?

This is unlikely. If the Lungs descend, the Kidneys are highly likely to grasp Lung Qi since that is where their Qi originates. The Kidneys give a pop as the Qi is received. If the Lungs descended Qi but the Kidneys did not to receive the Qi, you would feel the downward vector under your fingers but the pop would be absent.

How can I tell whether the Kidneys are exhibiting a false weakness?

The Kidneys get their Yang by grasping Qi from the Lungs as the Lungs descend it. If the Lungs don't descend, the weakness you feel in the Kidneys might not be weakness at all. Address the Lungs, generate descension there and then re-examine the Kidney pulse.

If I find a tight quality in at the moderate level of the chi position what organ should I consider?

The Bladder, Pericardium and Triple Heater can all show up in the chi positions. In some texts, the intestines are said to be present.

What does it mean if the Kidney pulse becomes tight as I explain to my patient that the Kidney pulse enables us to see deep into the constitution?

Chi, as in the chi position, means pattern but chi also means ten cun. So we're looking very deeply. If you ask about what you think might be suppressed in that pulse and it becomes tight, there might be trauma in the patient's history. Our job then, through treatment of the channels, becomes helping the patient come to terms with that trauma and surpass its constriction on the Jing-Essence, on the expression of Destiny. Healing is not to prevent challenges or dying, but to free the person from the constraints during the passage of living. The constraints on the actual passage, the actual unfolding of the Jing-Essence, show in the chi pulse.

I feel a strongly floating pulse in the Kidney Yang position. Also, as I was measuring the Lung to Kidney vector and felt the Qi go the other way, it felt as though it was surging upward. What can it mean?

This is an unusual pulse and can be found in cases of anemia, especially in women, as Kidney Yang moves up to the chest to help in the production of Blood. It is not a Triple Heater pulse.

QUESTIONS ABOUT TRIPLE HEATER

What kinds of Western medical conditions can relate to the Triple Heater pulse when there is no support offered the Triple Heater by the deep and moderate levels of the right chi?

If the right chi position is very rapid, floating and empty and there is no support from the moderate and deep levels, latency of pathology has been lost. Fire toxins have been freed from latency. The patient may have a pre-cancerous condition, AIDS, metastasized cancer, extreme damp accumulation, ascites, edema, swellings, etc.

If there is no Triple Heater pulse, does it mean conclusively that there is no fire toxin issue present?

No. You can have fire toxins that are spreading and moving within the Zang Fu without having a Triple Heater pulse. If the Triple Heater pulse appears, it means that either the person is very strong and is confident that an attempt at eradication may succeed, or the person is still containing the Heat (inflammation) which is still producing fire toxins (free radicals) and the condition cannot be cleared even though an attempt is being made. The Triple Heater pulse could also indicate the body has become so saturated with a pathogen that the fire toxins are leaking out of the Jing. The Triple Heater pulse does not appear if the fire toxins have leaked and the body does not have sufficient Qi to clear them. So a significant spreading (metastasis) of fire toxins can be occurring and yet the body might show no Triple Heater pulse.

How can I tell the difference between a Triple Heater pulse and a Tai Yang Sinew pulse?

The Triple Heater pulse floats from the deep level. If you engage the deep level of the chi position (usually on the right, but it is possible, though rarely, to find it on the left) and you allow your finger slowly to go to the superficial level, finding it rapid the entire time, and it follows your finger, presenting pressure to your finger as you lift it up above one bean of pressure, perhaps even projecting outside the confines of the skin, you have found a Triple Heater pulse. This is a marker of an interior condition, venting. If the pulse is simply tight and isolated in the superficial level and has no palpable connection to the deep (or moderate) level in that you didn't feel it originating at a deeper level and floating up there, you have found a Sinew pulse. The condition is one of the exterior.

Can a Triple Heater pulse be leathery or scattered?

Yes. If it is scattered it is either trying to bring pathology out, or it has little integrity. Assess which is the case by pressing back into the deep level to see how forceful and wide the pulse is.

How can I tell if there is metastasis happening?

Press down from the superficial to moderate level in the chi position. Determine whether there is strength underneath in the moderate level. If it lacks strength, the body is not trying to get rid of something; instead, the toxins are spreading. Bring the pathogen back into latency. If you are concerned about metastasis (autointoxication) you might consider the Eight Extra Channels or the Divergent Channels.

What is the diagnosis that relates to the Triple Heater pulse?

Fire toxins clearing from the Jing-Essence, or fire toxins moving from the Jing-Essence. The rest of the diagnosis would provide the detail about why this is happening (depletion of Fluids, Blood, Yin or Jing). Write it down, then calmly do your work.

Why do I feel that I am finding lots of Triple Heater pulses?

You're probably finding Yang Ming Sinew pulses which can be found on the right but are generally found on the left, or you're finding that Yang is escaping. Escaping Yang is common in our Yin deficient culture due to the excess consumption of coffee, hot spices, chocolate, alcohol, garlic and onion, and the failure to eat wet food and soups, go to sleep early and cultivate health. Read the description of the Triple Heater pulse carefully (page 195). It is not common in the general population.

The Complement Channels perform the common function of keeping pathology away from the Zang Fu. A pathogen will first encounter the Sinew Channels which create sneezes, sweat, coughing, vomiting, diarrhea or frequent urination to release the pathogen. They can also create tightness to hold the pathogen in the exterior until enough resources have been gathered to release it.

APPENDIX III

HOW TO USE THIS BOOK

Readers of this book probably fall somewhere on a continuum. At one end of the continuum are experienced practitioners who are skilled in their method of pulse taking and curious about the body of knowledge shared here. At the other end are students and practitioners who feel their pulse taking abilities never properly developed. This book is dense and comprehensive, but it need not be daunting. Studying pulses requires a strategy, an order. Here are some suggestions for organizing the study of pulses. I suggest working your way through this list at a comfortable pace. Some people might take years to complete it, others months. Ideally, become confident with each step before moving to the next. By the end, you will feel remarkably comfortable with pulses. If you are a practitioner you might consider taking pulses as you normally would, but every week adding one of these steps.

1. Study the theory of the connection you are making by taking the pulse, in Chapter One. Prepare your mind for the deep encounter you are going to develop.

2. Become very comfortable with locating the pulse positions on the wrist. Try it on your friends, family, patients, fellow students. Don't get into diagnosis yet, just get orientated. Locate LU-9. Make sure you can feel the Kidney pulse in most of the people.

3. When confident with step 2, practice the exercise that allows you to feel the tremendous depth available for analysis in the pulse, on page 59. Practice it on all your test people. Keep doing it until you feel in awe of the amount of space the pulse region occupies.

4. Study the five parameters in Chapter Two. Spend a period simply practicing registering the height/depth of the pulse. Cultivate ease while in contact with the pulses and moving through its depths. Start by simply resting your fingers on the pulses. Move between one bean (barely touching the pulse) to 15 beans (pressing into the bone) and then move between three beans, nine beans and 12 beans of pressure. Keep going back and forth between the three levels until you feel comfortable identifying them. Note how some pulses will come up to the Wei level and others will not protrude above the Yuan level.

5. Study the following qualities: weak, full, tight, wiry, thin, choppy, narrow, slippery, moving, superficial and floating. Practice finding these qualities.

6. Spend time finding tight pulses. Tight pulses feel as though they are being pressed in at the sides. The top of the pulse pushes up into your finger as a result. Then look for tight pulses

in all three levels in all positions. Then spend time practicing finding choppy pulses.

7. Practice finding slippery pulses. Slippery pulses feel as though they have no consonant-like definition at the beginning of the beat. Look for slippery pulses especially in Lung, Spleen, Liver and Kidney positions.

8. Practice finding superficial pulses. When approaching the pulse, very lightly touch your finger to the pulse at about one bean of pressure. A Sinew pulse is tight, superficial and pushes up against your finger. Look in all six finger positions for Sinew pulses.

9. Spend a period simply registering the width of the pulses in each position at each of the three levels. This is a total of nine positions. Hopefully Kidney pulses will generally be found only at the deep level and be quite wide on the left.

10. Spend a period simply registering the length of each of the pulses.

11. Spend a period measuring the tempos of the cun, guan and chi positions. Then practice finding the tempos at each of their three levels. Start without referencing the breath at all. Just sit with the pulses and see if one pulse is vibrating faster than the others. Explore the Wei, Ying and Yuan levels. Very often, the degree of rapidity changes with the level. This tells you which channel or which organ has the Heat. When you feel confident in this, begin measuring the pulse against the breath. A normal pulse tempo is four beats per breath.

12. Study the concept of directionality in Chapter Four. Begin practicing directionality by determining whether the Spleen ascends to the Lungs (the Spleen to Lung vector). Place your fingers in the pulse neutral position. Press the cun and guan positions to nine beans and the chi position to 12 beans. Add a little more pressure to the Spleen finger while at the same time releasing a tiny bit of pressure from the cun position. If you felt a pop at the cun position, it means that the Spleen is ascending Qi to the Lungs.

13. Find that vector on your test population. Once you have that vector under your belt, the rest of the vectors follow. Add a new vector every so often until you are practicing them all.

14. Study probing pulses in Chapter 3. This will help refresh your knowledge of organ function and help you match that knowledge to what you can feel in the pulse. Practice probing pulses in the right wrist in your test people.

15. Practice probing pulses in the left wrist of your test people.

16. In your practice, be sure to take the pulses during and after each treatment to orientate yourself to the effects your treatments are having.

17. Gradually learn all the pulse qualities listed in Chapter Two.

18. Keep practicing. As in all aspects of Chinese Medicine, the learning never stops no matter how proficient you become in pulse taking.

Chinese Medicine is not linear. Rather, it tends to holographic. All things and anything can be in the pulses at once, but we can't perceive them all at once. Or, at least we can't note them all at once. The ideal transmission of pulse technique would be to simply sit, take pulses, and transmit the feeling of it. There's a way of learning that has no words, sitting with someone deeply experienced in pulses, who somehow transmits to another practitioner the intention to witness, to hear, to feel the invitation to the pulses to reveal what needs to be known. There's a feeling of being flexible in order to receive that information.

With all that in mind, writing a book on pulses is challenging. Such a book has to be linear in order to be clear, and yet the notion of the medicine transcending linear explanation must be present at all times. Nevertheless, it's my hope that after digesting this book, you are able to suspend the idea of sequential inquiry and engage in the experience of the vast ocean that is the pulse. Let the pulse speak to you. Allow it to reach up into your consciousness. Once there, the fruits of the study will enable you to decipher the possibilities the patient is presenting, in the intimate, limitless and unique world of their pulses.

APPENDIX IV

ENTITIC INVASIONS

A couple of years ago, my housekeeper, who is usually in robust health, complained about being unusually tired. I placed my hand on her right wrist and found that her pulses, which were normally remarkably clear, had become slippery but not slippery enough to explain the tiredness. As I put my fingers on the left pulses a sensation like a small electric shock pushed my index finger off the Heart pulse position. I felt as though my finger had been zapped. I told her that I thought she probably had an entity in her apartment and she immediately responded, "I knew it!". It turned out that she and her two year old daughter had just moved to a different apartment. Soon after moving they both seemed to have a cold that would neither settle in nor clear. After her treatment and her own treatment of their apartment, all was cleared, and when I next saw her the pulses were back to her normal.

Usually entities (gui) show up in the Heart pulse, but they can technically show in any pulse. The sensation on the finger is of unpleasantness, electricity, even repulsion, as though it were pushing you off the skin. Your finger simply wants to be free of the pulse.

If you find an unusual situation where the pulse is floating in the cun and chi positions and at the same time there is nothing superficial or deep in the guan position, an entity is likely present. When all the pulses are superficial and there are no other pulses palpable including hidden pulses, there may be an entity present, according to the *Mai Jing*.

Entities can also show up as Qiao pulses after the death of someone close. The Yang Qiao pulse arises when there is a death and the patient's home is possessed. The Yin Qiao pulse also arises when there is a death and the patient is possessed. Treat the Qiaos in these cases, before moving on perhaps to Yin Wei Mai.

The full gamut of treatments for entitic invasions is extensive and beyond the scope of this book, but because I am describing the pulses of invasion, here is the principal treatment: Take five half-inch needles each with a loop on the end of their metal handle. Needle GV-26, LU-11 and SP-1 all perpendicularly. Carefully moxa both LU-11's and SP-1's with pole moxa until they feel to the patient as though they are tingling. Ask the patient to consciously push the energy of the entity off their body. (I ask them to push the energy off through their eyes while concentrating on one spot on the ceiling. This part is not classical Chinese, but it is ancient nonetheless.) Leave the room for a few minutes. Return and remove the needles. Open the window and immediately close it. Clap your hands around the room. Declare the patient and the room free of the entity. The patient should eat something as soon as possible.

ENTITIES AND THE PRACTITIONER

The practitioner has the responsibility to remain clear of entities through cultivation. This is a lengthy subject and beyond the scope of this book. If you feel that you are encountering an entity in the treatment room, it is important to view it simply as an energy that has no significance to you whatsoever. If even then you feel something come into your hand, clench your jaw and push it back to the patient. I have not had to do this in all my years of practice. It is sufficient to simply observe the energy no matter how it appears, and register that it is not yours.

APPENDIX V

INTUITION AND THE PULSES

Interacting with someone at their pulses is surprisingly intimate. The patient is allowing you to peer even into their Yuan level. They're allowing you to see more of them than any person would allow a friend to see. And at the same time, they're a bit mystified. They're marveling that this ancient medicine has tools which seem simple and nearly magical in their capacity. They might be habitually hiding something, but they're offering their wrist anyway.

For practitioners who are very sensitive it's often possible to feel that a diagnosis is coming through direct understanding—an intuition that's keenly honed. Perhaps a practitioner has a natural gift or an ability beyond the scope of acupuncture training. Any such talent is usable in such an encounter for the benefit of the patient. Indeed, so much information is available and must be sorted through: where to begin, where the patient's intention is focused, their signs and symptoms, their personality, their will-power, their expectations, their history. So many clinical decisions need to be made that intuition is one of our most indispensable tools.

However, at all times intuition must be supported by clear actual findings in the pulses. For those less experienced, it might be useful to imagine that if Wang Shu He were visiting, you would be able to say to him, "As I press into this position at this level, I get a strong sense of this quality. Don't you agree?" To be responsible in medicine, the findings of your intuition must line up with your findings in the five parameters of the pulse.

Chinese medicine includes many modes of thinking, including the highly intuitive, but at all times it resonates with demonstrable signs in the pulses that could be shared with others, that can be described and justified within the vast complexities of the classical teachings. Intuition can be an integral part of the diagnostic process but it arises from knowledge and must be responsible to the presentation of the pulses, however subtle.

RECOMMENDED READING

Dr Jeffrey Yuen, oral transmission. A primary source of oral transmission of Classical Chinese Medicine at an international level is Jeffrey Yuen, the 88th generation of his Taoist lineage: *Yu Ching Huang Lao Pai*, (Jade Purity School, Yellow Emperor/Lao Tzu sect); 26th generation of *Chuan Chen Lung Men Pai* (Complete Reality School, Dragon Gate Sect).

William Morris and Li Sheng-qing, *Li Shi-Zhen's Pulse Studies, An Illustrated Guide* (Beijing: People's Medical Publishing House, 2011).

Huang-Fu Mi, *The Systematic Classic of Acupuncture and Moxibustion* (Boulder: Blue Poppy Press, 1993).

Li Shi Zhen, *Pulse Diagnosis* (Brookline: Paradigm Publications, 1985).

Maoshing Ni, *The Yellow Emperor's Classic of Medicine* (Boston: Shambhala, 1995).

Paul Unschuld, translator, *Nan Ching, Classic of Difficult Issues* (Berkeley: University of California Press, 1986).

Paul Unschuld, general editor and translator, Hermann Tessenow, translator, *Huang Di Nei Jing Su Wen: An Annotated Translation of Huang Di's Inner Classic* (Berkeley: University of California Press, 2011).

Wang Shu-He, and Shou-Zhong, Yang, *The Pulse Classic, A Translation of the Mai Jing*, (Boulder: Blue Poppy, 1997).

Wu Jing-Nuan, translator, *Ling Shu or The Spiritual Pivot* (Honolulu: University of Hawaii Press, 1993).

Nelson Liansheng Wu, Andrew Qi Wu, translators, *Yellow Emperor's Canon Internal Medicine*, (Beijing: China Science and Technology Press, 1999).

Zhang, Ye, Wiseman, Mitchell, Feng, *Shang Han Lun, On Cold Damage*, (Brookline: Paradigm, 1999).

Leon I. Hammer, *Chinese Pulse Diagnosis: A Contemporary Approach* (Seattle: Eastland Press, 2005).

INDEX

ABOUT THE AUTHOR

Ann Cecil-Sterman, MS, L.Ac, is the author of the widely acclaimed book, *Advanced Acupuncture: A Clinic Manual*, a required text in many acupuncture schools in the United States. She travels all over the world to teach the application and methodology of the Complement Channels, the art of pulse diagnosis, and the use of food as medicine. For many years she taught Advanced Clinical Observation and was a senior clinic supervisor at the school of acupuncture founded by Dr Jeffrey Yuen in 1997 in New York City. She is a long-time student of Dr Yuen, having extensively studied acupuncture, diet, Chinese medical history, herbs, qigong, essential oils, stones and philosophy with him across North America. She also studied pulses and the Complementary Channels with Dr Sheila George. Ann was Director of the Classical Wellness Center in Manhattan where for many years she practiced and taught classes on advanced diagnosis and the theory and application of Classical Chinese Medicine. Currently, her patients—children and adults of all ages—come from all over the world, working through illnesses or on personal cultivation. Ann's practice features the Complement Channels of acupuncture: the Sinew, Luo, Divergent and Eight Extraordinary Channels, and is augmented with Classical Chinese dietary therapeutic guidance. She lives in Manhattan with her husband and two children.

ABOUT THE DESIGNER

Cody Dodo, MS, L.Ac, studied acupuncture under the tutelage of Dr Jeffrey Yuen at the Swedish Institute in New York. He also completed advanced studies with Dr Yuen in acupuncture and Chinese nutritional therapy. He lectures about Chinese Medicine in New York, and internationally. Prior to his pursuit of acupuncture, Cody had a long career as a graphic designer in the publishing industry. By combining his Chinese medical knowledge with his visual sensibility, Cody is able to convey the author's ideas with clear and simple diagrams and design. He also designed the author's first book, *Advanced Acupuncture: A Clinic Manual*. He has a private practice in Manhattan, teaches Classical Acupuncture internationally, and lives with his wife in Brooklyn.

Printed in the USA
CPSIA information can be obtained
at www.ICGtesting.com
LVHW071826161023
761236LV00014B/242